Bone Marrow Transplantation and Other Treatment after Radiation Injury

Bone Marrow Transplantation and Other Treatment after Radiation Injury

A review prepared for the Commission of the European Communities, Directorate-General Research, Science and Education (Biology-Medical Research)

H. Balner M.D.

Martinus Nijhoff Medical Division - The Hague 1977
for
The Commission of the European Communities

Publication arranged by

Commission of the European Communities, Directorate-General Scientific and Technical Information and Information Management, Luxembourg

EUR 5884e

ISBN   978-90-247-2056-9   ISBN   978-94-010-1113-6   (eBook)
DOI   10.1007/978-94-010-1113-6

Abstract

This review deals mainly with current concepts about bone marrow transplantation as therapy for serious radiation injury. Such injury can be classified according to the following broadly defined dose ranges: (1) the supralethal range, leading mainly to the cerebral and intestinal syndromes; (2) the potentially lethal or therapeutic range which causes the bone marrow syndrome, and (3) the sublethal range which rarely leads to injury requiring therapy. The bone marrow syndrome of man and animals is discussed in detail. The optimal therapy for this syndrome is bone marrow transplantation in conjunction with conventional supportive treatment. The principal complications of such therapy are Graft versus Host Disease and a slow recovery of the recipient's immune system.

Concerted research activities in a number of institutions have led to considerable progress in the field of bone marrow transplantation. Improved donor selection, new techniques for stem-cell separation and preservation, as well as effective barrier-nursing and antibiotic decontamination, have made bone marrow transplantation an accepted therapy for marrow depression, including the aplasia caused by excessive exposure to radiation. The review also contains a number of guidelines for the handling of serious radiation accidents.

Dr. H. Balner is a staff member of the Commission of the European Communities, Directorate – General Research, Science and Education (Biology – Medical Research).
He is at present Director of the Primate Center – TNO, Rijswijk (ZH), The Netherlands.

Table of contents

1. Introduction

Acute radiation injury in man has been amply reviewed in the past decades (1-8). Information for those reviews was mainly derived from the Hiroshima and Nagasaki experience (3), from radiation accidents as a consequence of testing nuclear weapons and the application of nuclear energy (9-13) and from the intentional irradiation of patients, mostly for the treatment of malignancies and/or as conditioning for transplantation (14-20). Further, a large body of data derived from animal experimentation has led to cautious extrapolations to the human situation (14).

An elaborate review dealing with early somatic effects of radiation in man was published by UNSCEAR[a] in 1962 (2). It was supplemented in 1969 with a similar document dealing mostly with radiation-induced chromosome aberrations, the effects of radiation on the nervous system and, radio-active contamination of the environment by nuclear testing (21). In a more recent UNSCEAR report (1972) the main topics were genetic effects, carcinogenesis and effects of radiation on the immune response (22). The early effects of radiation in man were also expertly and comprehensively reviewed in a report by the United States National Research Council in 1967 (23).

In the past decade the scientific interpretations of nearly all aspects of radiation injury to man have not undergone significant changes. There is one aspect, however, which has shown dynamic progress and can be expected to change even more dramatically in the coming years, namely the replacement of hemopoietic tissue following radiation accidents in the potentially lethal dose range[b]. Fortunately, the number of radiation casualties which required such bone marrow transplantations has been minimal, up to now. However, in view of the more widespread application of nuclear energy and the growing intensity of nuclear research, it is not unreasonable to expect an increasing number of radiation accidents and thus a growing need for effective bone marrow transplantation in man. Needless to mention that demands for such therapy could take on very large proportions in the case of

----

[a] United Nations Scientific Committee on the Effects of Atomic Radiation

[b] The expression "potentially lethal" relates to external radiation doses which can have fatal consequences, in contrast to doses defined as sublethal which are never fatal and those defined as supralethal, which always have a fatal outcome (see later, table I).

1

nuclear warfare. However, in such a disastrous event, the majority of the casualties would suffer from blast injuries and burns or from the delayed effects of radio-active fallout rather than from acute overexposure which could be remedied by bone marrow transplantation. Moreover, the transplantation of bone marrow (as practised today) still requires meticulous preparations, a close collaboration of numerous specialists and highly specialized medical facilities (see section 5 of this review). The chaotic situation and disruption of normal medical care which is likely to occur in nuclear warfare, can hardly be expected to provide favorable circumstances for bone marrow transplantation.

The aim of this document is to review the current therapeutic possibilities for early effects of radiation injury to man and animals. Fundamental radiobiological issues will be dealt with in a cursory fashion, since they have not changed significantly since the appearance of the elaborate reviews mentioned earlier (2, 21, 22, 24). However, for the clinically oriented reader, certain fundamentals of radiobiology and a schematic classification of the most common types of radiation injury will be briefly reviewed in sections 2 and 3 of this document.

2. Biological effects of radiation

This is obviously not the place for a detailed discussion of the various types of radiation, their sources and the factors which influence their biological effect. Those subjects have been repeatedly reviewed in great detail (25, 26). Only the physical and biological factors which have a bearing on the clinical and experimental data to be described in sections 3 and 4, will be briefly discussed in the following paragraphs.

PHYSICAL FACTORS

An important characteristic of ionizing radiation is the localized release of a relatively large amount of energy, resulting in ionization of atoms and breakage of chemical bonds. Clusters of ion pairs are formed along a particle track and their spatial distribution is an important factor in determining the biological effectiveness. The density of clusters formed depends on the amount of energy deposited per unit track length, a quantity usually referred to as LET or Linear Energy Transfer (27, 28). When radiation doses are mentioned in this review without specification, acute single doses of low LET radiation are meant. It concerns so-called conventional high-intensity radiation, usually administered by common clinical X-ray machines (200 - 300 kVp) or gamma sources such as cobalt (^{60}Co) and caesium (^{137}Cs). Because of repair mechanisms after radiation damage (29), dose rate and dose fractionation are of great importance in determining the biological effect.

In general, the efficiency of a type of radiation to produce a certain effect in a biological system varies with LET. With increasing LET, an increase in relative biological effectiveness or RBE is also observed. The RBE can be defined as the inverse ratio of the dose of a standard radiation (usually 250 kVp X-rays) to the dose of the tested radiation required to produce the same biological effect under the same conditions. The RBE is not constant; it may vary with cell type, tissue, observed endpoint, etc. Reviews on this subject have been published (22, 25).

The most important single physical factor determining acute radiation damage, is the absorbed dose. The early radiation effects to be discussed, require a relatively high radiation dose, are strongly dose-rate dependent and show distinct dose thresholds. Moreover, the severity of symptoms is related to increasing doses in a non-linear fashion (23). In the framework of this review, detailed information about the methods to calculate absorbed doses, can obviously not be given. Suffice it to state, that the doses referred to will mostly be expressed in rad (absorbed dose) rather than in R (Roentgens) at the surface or R as midline dose in air[a].

In view of repair mechanisms after radiation damage (29), dose rate and dose fractionation are of great importance in determining the biological effect. However, since the early radiation effects to be discussed are mostly the consequence of acute or "high-intensity" radiation (see above), we shall refrain from giving details about protraction or fractionation of radiation. A few examples of the considerable influence of dose fractionation on a particular effect will be given when discussing local radiation of the skin and certain other tissues (see pages 10 - 12).

The spatial distribution of radiation is also a rather important parameter when assessing the radiation damage to be expected. The consequences of irradiating only certain anatomical regions or fractions of the total body, the influence of penetration and distribution of the radiation, etc., have been considered in numerous reports (2, 21, 22). The variation in spatial distribution of radiation received in accidents is virtually unlimited and data on distribution patterns are often vague, even after meticulous reconstruction of an accident (15). In order to facilitate the determination of dose response relationships for injuries in radiation accidents, some authors have proposed to express the dose as the absorbed dose (rad) in a 26 cm diameter sphere of tissue in the epigastric region, the most sensitive region with regard to "prodromal" symptoms (see later). When applying total body irradiation in animal experimentation and in cases of intentional radiation of patients prior to bone marrow transplantation, the spatial distribution of the dose is usually as homogeneous as possible.

----

[a] The new internationally accepted unit of absorbed dose, as defined in the "Système Internationale d'Unités" (S.I. units), is the gray (1 Gy = 1 J/kg). However, for the time being the rad is still accepted as unit of radiation dose (100 rad = 1 Gy).

4

The famous law of Bergonie and Tribondeau was formulated in 1906 and deals with the radiosensitivity of cells and tissues (30). It proclaims that the most radiosensitive cells are those which are least differentiated and have the highest mitotic rate. Since then, decades of experimental radio-biology have largely confirmed that ancient postulate. The most radiosensitive tissues of the mammalian organism (with cell death taken as endpoint) are indeed those with a high mitotic rate[a]: hemopoietic tissue, germinal epithelium, intestinal lining, epithelium of cutaneous appendages, etc. By the same criteria, the least sensitive cells are the highly differentiated parenchymal cells of organs, nerve cells, osteocytes, etc., all of which show low mitotic activity in vivo. In cell culture studies, however, survival curves of irradiated mammalian cells proved that many different cell types, including tumor cells, show only a limited variation in radiosensitivity (26). Thus, a parenchymal kidney cell with a slow growth rate in vivo is considered radioresistant, while the same cell type, once it acquires a high growth rate in vitro, turns out to be as radiosensitive as any other rapidly proliferating cell. In spite of this seeming discrepancy, the division of cells or tissues into radiosensitive and resistant ones, is quite convenient. For example, after total body radiation in the lethal dose range, the most disturbing early effects are clearly a consequence of immediate damage to the critical, radiosensitive tissues such as hemopoietic stem cells and intestinal epithelium (see later). In the context of this review the intricate and controversial fundamental issue of cellular radio-sensitivity needs no further discussion. Interested readers are referred to the abundant literature existing about this subject (31, 32).

Another interesting and biologically important issue is the individual resistance to radiation injury. When discussing the LD_{50} for the "bone marrow syndrome" (page 23), it will be shown that various animal species display a limited but distinct difference in their response to total body radiation (TBR). Interestingly, such differences are also observed when

----

[a]Lymphocytes may be the only major exception to this rule: they are highly radiosensitive in spite of slow renewal characteristics. This has been attributed to the so-called interphase death (14).

studying the effect on individuals of the same species or even the same inbred rodent strain[a]. It is well documented that the presence of certain pathogens in laboratory animals can have a significant influence on LD_{50} values for TBR (14) and that the LD_{50} value for germfree animals is somewhat higher than that for conventional animals of the same strain or species (33). However, factors not specifically related to resistance against invading microorganisms, may also contribute to the radiosensitivity of an animal. These factors are likely to include the general physical condition of an individual, the nutritional state and possibly the regenerative capacity of certain vital tissues. It is obvious that these comparatively minor individual differences in radiosensitivity will cease to play a decisive role in the "supralethal" dose range of total body radiation.

----

[a] Animals belonging to a particular inbred strain are, with regard to genetic similarity, comparable to monozygotic twins in humans.

3. Schematic classification of radiation injury

Radiation injury occurs at the time of exposure. The visible or measurable effects on an organism are revealed as signs or symptoms occurring after a certain latent period. Groups of symptoms are sometimes called syndromes or diseases (e.g. "radiation sickness"). For our further discussions it might be helpful to recapitulate briefly the major types of radiation injury and mention the factors which may influence their time of appearance and severity.

Injuries can be localized i.e. affecting only those tissues or organs which have received a sufficiently high dose to cause detectable lesions. In man, most examples are found in the radiotherapy of tumors where circumscribed areas are usually irradiated, and in a few radiation accidents (34-36). In experimental work, localized irradiation has been applied on a large scale to study injuries after exposure of certain parts of an animal's body (shielding of other parts of the body is usually required). Localized irradiation is not lethal unless vital organs (brain, heart, esophagus, lung, gut) receive doses in the "supralethal" range which, by definition, preclude recovery (see below). The injury is said to be generalized if the entire or nearly the entire body has been exposed. Obviously, ensuing signs and symptoms again depend on factors such as radiation dose, quality, dose-rate, distribution, etc. A conventional classification of these injuries, graded according to severity, is presented on pages 13 to 16. Although regional radiation can also be subdivided into dose ranges which can have a lethal effect or not, the conventional classification into supralethal, (potentially) lethal, and sublethal ranges usually refers to total-body radiation (TBR). Table I gives a highly schematic presentation of these ranges and their most common signs and symptoms in man. It can be seen that what is commonly designated as the lethal range has been subdivided into one which is inevitably lethal or supralethal (> 1000 rad) and a "potentially" lethal range of between 200 and 1000 rad. This arbitrary subdivision is based on the consideration that radiation doses in the potentially lethal range cause injuries which are sometimes amenable to effective therapy, while lesions caused by doses in the supralethal range are not.

TABLE I

TOTAL BODY RADIATION IN MAN: SCHEMATIC CLASSIFICATION OF DOSE RANGES, SYMPTOMS, THERAPY AND OUTCOME[a]

| Exposure[b] (high intensity, conventional X-ray or γ-radiation) | | Prodromal Symptoms | | Clinical Characteristics | | | Possible Therapy, Clinical Course and Outcome | | | | | |
dose (range)	dose (rad)	nausea, vomiting, etc. incidence	delay in appearance	organ systems mainly involved	characteristic symptoms	critical period after exposure	therapy	time until recovery	prognosis	lethality	if injury is fatal: death occurring within	usual cause of death
lethal or "supralethal" (>1000 rad)	>5000	100%	minutes	central nervous and cardiovascular (CEREBRAL SYNDROME)	- cramps - tremor - ataxia - lethargy - impaired vision - coma	1-48 hours	palliative	--	hopeless	100%	1-48 hours	cerebral edema and/or cardiovascular decompensation
	1000-1500	100%	30 min.	gastrointestinal (INTESTINAL SYNDROME)	- diarrhea - fever - electrolytic imbalance	3-14 days	palliative	--	very poor	90-100%	2 weeks	enterocolitis shock
potentially lethal or therapeutic lethal (200-1000 rad)	500-1000	100%	1 hour	blood forming tissues (BONE MARROW SYNDROME)	- thrombopenia - leucopenia - hemorrhages - infections - epilation (>300 rad)	2-6 weeks	- optimal care (isolation, antibiotics, fluids etc.) - transfusions of leucocytes, platelets - bone marrow transplantation	weeks, months, years	uncertain (depending on success of therapy)	0-90%	weeks or months	hemorrhages, infections
	200-500	100% (>300 rad)	2 hours									
sublethal (0-200 rad)	100-200	50% (>200 rad) 5% (>100 rad)	3 hours	blood forming tissues	mild leucopenia and thrombopenia	--	observation, tranquilization	several weeks	excellent	--	--	--
	0-100	--	--	--	--	--	tranquilization	--	excellent	--	--	--

a) based on pooled data from accidental and therapeutic radiation of man and extrapolation of experimental animal data

b) high intensity, conventional X-ray or γ-radiation as defined in text, page 3

Adapted from a Report of the General Secretary of the UN to the General Assembly of the UN; document A/6858 10 October 1967.

Early effects can be observed within a few minutes after exposure but
the majority of early signs and symptoms occurs within the first weeks and
up to day 60. The latter limit has been chosen as an arbitrary (but reasonable) cut-off point, since symptoms which fail to appear within 60 days will
usually not reveal themselves until months or years later (23). Late effects
are those occurring months or years after exposure. They include genetic
effects, life shortening, oncogenesis, and numerous degenerative changes in
various tissues and organs and have been extensively described (22). Since
this review is concerned with replacement therapy of hemopoietic tissue
(bone marrow transplantation) and since such therapy is not known to be
beneficial for late effects of radiation, the subsequent classification of
injuries deals with early somatic effects only.

LOCALIZED EFFECTS

As briefly indicated, radiation injury can be localized, i.e. affecting
only those tissues or organs which have received a sufficiently high dose to
cause detectable lesions. In man, most examples of localized effects can be
seen as a consequence of the radiotherapy of tumors where circumscribed
areas are usually irradiated, and as a result of radiation accidents (34,
35, 36).

-    Irradiation of the head region. One can argue whether injury of the
     head and brain should be considered a regional effect, since total body
     radiation in the supralethal dose range produces the same acute signs
     and symptoms. In any case, numerous experiments have shown that inten-
     sive radiation of the head only, will cause death within minutes or
     hours (37, 38). The onset of symptoms and the survival time are
     obviously related to the dose, quality, and intensity of the radiation.
     Doses of 100,000 - 200,000 rad kill almost instantly, probably by des-
     truction of medullary centers (39). Doses between 5000 and 100,000 rad
     produce symptoms mainly associated with damage to the central nervous
     system and death follows within one or two days. In monkeys, electro-
     encephalographic changes, without subsequent death, have been observed
     after doses of a few thousand rad of gamma-radiation given to the head
     region (40). The lowest radiation doses to the head region which pro-

9

duced lethal injury were described in the early sixties: death occurred within 2 weeks after X-ray doses of 1500 rad of the head, jaw or tongue of mice (41) and rats (42). The mechanism of these fatalities is probably due to interference with normal food-intake (due to infected ulcers of the tongue), rather than to a specific effect on the central nervous system (14). In similar experiments, dogs withstood doses of 1750 rad to the head region (43). A further description of signs and symptoms occurring after radiation injury to the brain will be discussed under "generalized effects".

- Irradiation of the abdominal region. As already indicated, the gastrointestinal syndrome is produced mainly by injury to the highly radiosensitive epithelial lining of the intestine. In most species, it occurs at absorbed doses in the "supralethal" dose range (Table I). Symptomwise, it makes little difference whether the dose is given as local irradiation to the abdominal region, as irradiation of a large (separated) bowel segment, or as total body radiation (44-47). Time of onset and severity of the syndrome again depend (within certain limits) on dose, dose-rate and quality of the radiation. After lethal doses, the immediate cause of death is fluid and electrolyte depletion which can be somewhat mitigated by resection of the injured bowel segment or by shielding of small portions of the duodenum or the ileum, not the coecum. Unlike in the shielding of part of the bone marrow (see later), the observed protection is probably due to local restoration of part of the small bowel function and not to an accelerated general repopulation of the intestinal epithelium (48). Below certain critical doses (in mammals mostly around 1000 rad), survival can also be prolonged by massive replacement of fluids and electrolytes (14, 49).

- Irradiation of the skin. While most available data for regional radiation injury of brain and gut are derived from animal experimentation, effects of localized radiation of the skin have been primarily studied in man. An excellent review of the subject was published in 1967 by the Space Science Board of the United States National Research Council (23). The bulk of data regarding the reactions of human skin to radiation are derived from clinical radiotherapy. Levels of early skin responses are, in order of increasing severity, designated as: erythema, dry desquamation, moist desquamation, sloughing of skin layers and chronic

10

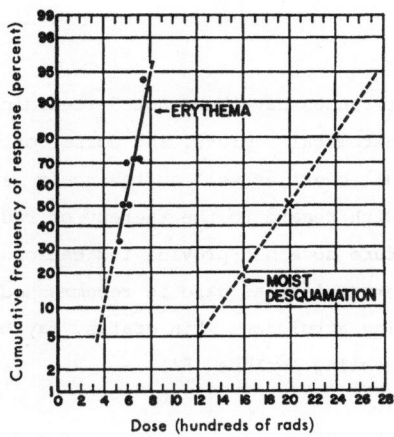

Fig. 1 Dose-frequency relationship of minimal erythema (135) and
moist desquamation (clinical tolerance response) for acute
exposure to 200 kVp X-rays.
Adapted from a figure which appeared in ref. 23 (page 63).

ulceration. Restoration of the skin to near-normal conditions occurs in
all categories, except the chronic ulceration stage. Yet, permanently
visable changes may remain even after dry desquamation. Fig. 1 provides
a graphic presentation of the dose-frequency relationship for erythema
versus moist desquamation of the human skin (the dose response curve
for dry desquamation should be between the two lines depicted in the
figure). A schematic presentation of the principal skin lesions, the
radiation doses which produce them (in 50 % of cases), and the long-
term consequences, are summarized in table II.

TABLE II

ESTIMATED RELATIONSHIP BETWEEN ACUTE·EXPOSURE TO X-RAYS AND SKIN INJURY IN MAN[a]

symptoms	approx. dose producing effect[b] in 50 % of cases	long term consequences	therapy
erythema	600 rad	none	unnecessary
dry desquamation	1200 rad	minor, mostly cosmetic	routine dermatological care and dressings; possibly reconstructive surgery (skin transpl.)
moist desquamation sloughing and chronic ulceration	2000 rad	severe chronic skin lesions	

[a] derived from data presented in ref. 23

[b] single exposure, "conventional" 200 kVp X-rays, rate 30 rad/min. or more

Interesting differences have been noted regarding the sensitivity of various exposed anatomical regions. The dorsae of the hands and feet (in particular the nail beds) as well as the scalp seem to be rather sensitive (23, 50). With regard to the therapy of radiation injury to the skin, the literature does not provide indications for specific treatment. Routine dermatological care is recommended and reconstructive surgery, including autologous skin grafts, may be indicated in cases of chronic, disabling lesions (51).

- Other localized effects. Extremely high doses of radiation to any part of the body will obviously result in early effects specific for the particular tissue or organ (heart, kidney, lung, esophagus, muscle, eyes, etc.). However, such localized injuries usually do not occur without simultaneous lesions to other vital organs.

  Isolated early effects have been described for the male gonads; radiation effects on spermatogonia (early precursors or stem cells of the spermatozoa) can be seen histologically within 3-6 hours after exposure. This effect is reflected some 50-70 days later as a drop in the sperm count, often associated with reduced fertility. The approximate dose/response relation for single doses of conventional high-intensity irradiation has been described (2) as follows: ∼ 150 rad induces temporary subfertility; ∼ 250 rad, temporary sterility for 1-2 years; 500-600 rad, temporary or permanent sterility; ∼ 800 rad, permanent sterility in virtually all cases. The genetic effects of radiation injury to the germinal tissue have been extensively reviewed elsewhere (22).

GENERALIZED EFFECTS

Generalized effects are mostly produced by intentional or accidental exposure of the individual to an extraneous radiation source (total body radiation or TBR), occasionally by intentional or accidental ingestion of radioactive material. For humans, the sources of information are mainly the clinical use of X- or gamma rays (treatment of malignancies and conditioning for transplantation), accidental exposure of workers in the nuclear indus-

12

try, and - of course - the data provided by studies on victims of nuclear explosions or their fallout. Table III presents a schematic listing of the major accidents of the past 3 decades and their clinical consequences. Detailed data regarding all accidents of the past decades, including the minor ones, have been published (52-57) while a permanent registry of all traceable radiation accidents is maintained in the U.S.A.[a].

Although still rather scarce, data obtained from the clinical application of total body irradiation are, as a whole, more reliable than those collected from accidental radiation of man. In the clinical cases, radiation quality, dose, dose distribution etc., are usually well-defined. However, in therapeutic cases of TBR, the interpretations may be complicated by the underlying disease and the additional treatment which is usually given. Clinical TBR at sublethal and median lethal dose levels has been performed mainly during the past two decades and in only a few selected centers. Indications were attempts to erradicate malignancies (mostly leukemias) and/or the conditioning of patients for bone marrow transplantation. In most cases conventional therapeutic X-ray machines or gamma-ray sources (^{60}Co, ^{137}Cs) were used. Detailed information regarding the clinical cases of TBR can be found in the appropriate literature. Some selected data will be presented in section 4 of this review, when the therapeutic potential of bone marrow transplantation after intentional or accidental radiation of humans is discussed (pages 43 to 54).

The bulk of information regarding the early generalized effects of total body radiation and its therapy clearly comes from animal experimentation. Most of the data were obtained with small rodents as experimental animals, but results which are probably most suitable for extrapolation to man have been obtained in experiments with dogs and rhesus monkeys. In principle, however, the symptomatology of the various radiation syndromes is similar for all mammalian species investigated. The following section describes those early syndromes. Whenever distinct differences are known to exist between the various species regarding the symptomatology of the radiation syndromes, this will be indicated in the text and in a few figures or tables.

----

[a] ERDA (Energy Research Developmental Administration), Div. of Biomedicine and Environmental Programs, Washington DC 20545, U.S.A.

TABLE III

PRINCIPAL RADIATION ACCIDENTS (1945 - 1975); SCHEMATIC LISTING OF EVENTS AND CONSEQUENCES

DESCRIPTION OF ACCIDENTS				RADIATION CONDITIONS		CLINICAL FINDINGS				
date	location	probable cause of accident	individuals exposed and/or injured	radiation quality and dose (estimates)	dose distribution	signs and symptoms	therapy if any	clinical course	probable cause of death (if fatal)	remarks
8-21-'45 and 5-21-'46	Los Alamos, New Mexico, USA. I and II	criticality	1	706 rad γ; 156 rad neutron	non-uniform	intestinal/hematological syndrome	symptomatic	death day 9	intestinal	severe epidermiolysis
			1	840 rad γ; 487 rad neutron	non-uniform	extensive burns, tachycardia	symptomatic	death day 25	fibrinous pericarditis	pre-existing heart condition; myocardema developed after accident, not clear whether this cond. was pre-existing
			1	407 rad γ; 41 rad neutron	mainly head, neck and chest	lethargy, somnolence	hardly any	recovery	-	radiation does not seem to have influenced patient's, excellent physical condition
			1	210 rad γ; 19 rad neutron	uniform	hematological symptoms (short duration)	-	favorable	-	-
			5	100 rad γ; 10 rad neutron	not mentioned	no clinically diagnosed injuries	-	-	-	-
6-2-'52	Argonne, Illinois, USA	criticality	4	190 rem, mixed 1/	not mentioned	no clinically diagnosed injuries	-	-	-	-
between '52 and '54	USSR	violation of operating rules of experimental reactor	1	300 rad, size 1	uniform	CNS , hematological syndrome	symptomatic	gradual improvement with complete recovery after 18 months	-	both cases have been described as "acute radiation disease"
			1	450 rad, size 1	uniform	CNS, intestinal and hematological syndrome	-	dramatic worsening of clinical condition day 10, followed by gradual improvement; recovery 18th month	-	
12-8-'53	Melbourne, Australia	60Co-capsule in pocket	1	no details given	mainly right leg	severe necrosis right leg	amputation right leg	recovery	-	-
6-16-'58	Oak Ridge, Y-12 plant, Tenn., USA	criticality	1	365 rad , mixed	uniform	intestinal/hematological syndrome, hair loss	symptomatic	recovery; discharge hospital day 44	-	-
			1	339 rad, mixed	uniform	mainly hematological syndrome	symptomatic	recovery; discharge hospital day 44	-	-
			1	327 rad, mixed	uniform	intestinal/hematological syndrome; hair loss	symptomatic	recovery; discharge hospital day 44	-	
			1	270 rad, mixed	uniform	hematological syndrome; infections	symptomatic	recovery; discharge hospital day 44	-	
			1	236 rad, mixed	uniform	hematological syndrome; hair loss	no specific treatment	recovery; discharge hospital day 44	-	
			3	68 rad, mixed	uniform	asymptomatic	-	-	-	3 cases were only hospitalized for observation
10-15-'58	Vinca, Yugoslavia	criticality	1	320 rad γ, 320 rad neutron	uniform	hematological/gastro-intestinal symptoms of ominous character	fetal liver, later bone marrow graft	death 5th week	intestinal invaginations plus massive hemorrhages	terminal jaundice; total absence of sperms at autopsy
			1	290 rad γ, 290 rad neutron	uniform	hematological gastrointestinal syndrome	bone marrow grafts (unrelated, adult donor) and symptomatic ther.	gradual improvement without complete recovery after 2 years	-	persisting azoospermia
			1	300 rad γ, 300 rad neutron	uniform				-	hypospermia
			1	250 rad γ, 250 rad neutron	uniform				-	serious menstrual disturbances
			1	210 rad γ, 210 rad neutron	uniform	same, though less severe symptoms	symptomatic	favorable	-	hypospermia
			1	175 rad γ, 175 rad neutron	uniform				-	
12-30-'58	Los Alamos, New Mexico, USA	criticality	1	3000 rad γ, 926 rad neutron	uniform	CNS (coma), gastro-intestinal and hemato-logical symptoms, cardiovascular shock	symptomatic	death after 35 hours	heart failure	acute myocarditis
			2	130 and 53 rad, mixed	uniform	asymptomatic	-	-	-	2 cases hospitalized for

Date / Location	Radiation source	No.	Uncertainty in estimated total dose	non-uniform	haematological symptoms / to lesser degree all or part of above symptoms	no specific therapy	outcome	cardiac / respiratory	retinal changes
6-8-'60 USSR	137Cs-source held against body (suicide)	1 / 2	± 1480 rad γ minimally exposed	non-uniform	asymptomatic	symptomatic	death day 18	severe emaciation	in one patient temporary quadriplegia
11-9-'60 USSR	radium bromide ingestion	1	2.03 millicuries (ingested)	non-uniform	gastrointestinal/haemato-logical syndrome	symptomatic	recovery	-	retained 100 microcuries
1-3-'61 Idaho Falls, Idaho, USA	explosion	3	In this case, dose is not important	not important	gastrointestinal/haemato-logical syndrome	symptomatic	-	blast injuries	-
1961 Fontenay aux Roses, France	explosion	9	minimally exposed	uniform	asymptomatic	-	-	-	members of rescue team
	explosion	1	no details given	no details given	injury arm	no details given	no details given	-	person "contaminated", more details not available
3-21-'62 Mexico City, Mexico	60Co-capsule found and stored in kitchen for almost 4 months	1	2940 - 5160 rem γ roughly estimated dose	non-uniform	gastrointestinal/haemato-logical syndrome + ulcer left thigh	symptomatic	death after about 5 weeks	combined cardiac / respiratory	autopsy not performed
		1	1959 - 2930 rem γ roughly estimated dose	non-uniform	CNS, gastrointestinal/haematological syndrome	symptomatic	death after about 4 months	heart arrest	at autopsy: multiple hemorrhages, bone marrow aplasia, massive tissue destruction
			1373 - 1872 rem γ roughly estimated dose	uniform	neuro-muscular/gastro-intestinal/haematologi-cal syndrome	symptomatic	death after about 5 months	Bronchopneumonia complicating bone marrow aplasia	at autopsy: multiple hemorrhages mainly in gastrointestinal tract and adrenals
		1	1518 - 2827 rem γ roughly estimated dose	uniform	mainly haematological syndrome; bleeding tendency	symptomatic	death after about 7 months	massive pulmonary hemorrhage with sub-sequent anoxia	at autopsy: severe bone marrow aplasia
		1	994 - 1716 rem γ roughly estimated dose	uniform	neuro-muscular/CNS, pneumonitis	no specific treatment	recovery	-	aspermia, testicular atrophy
4-7-'62 Hanford, Wash., USA	criticality	3	19 - 110 rem, mixed	uniform	asymptomatic	no treatment	-	-	significant increase in chromosome aberrations in circulating leucocytes
6-24-'64 Rhode Island, USA	criticality	1	8800 rad γ	uniform	CNS/gastrointestinal/haematological symptoms	no treatment	death after 49 hours	cardiovascular	admission to hospital diffi-cult because of unfounded fear for radioact. contamin
		2	100 rad γ	uniform	asymptomatic	-	-	-	
2-18-'65 Rockford, Illinois, USA	accelerator accident	1	300 - 240,000 rad γ	non-uniform	necrosis skin, muscles, nerves, bone	amputation R.extremities	"recovery"	-	-
12-30-'65 Mol, Belgium	criticality	1	200 rad γ, 400 rad γ, 3000 - 5000 rad γ	head, trunk, L.foot	gastrointestinal/haemato-logical symptoms; necrosis foot	symptomatic; amputation L. foot	recovery	-	-
10-4-'67 Gulf Company, Pittsburgh, Penn., USA	accelerator accident, failure of safety measures	1	400 - 2400 rad, mixed	mainly trunk	mainly haematological syndrome	bone marrow graft from identical twin brother	recovery	-	bone marrow graft considered life-saving
		1	400 - 700 rad, mixed	mainly extremities	necrosis of all extremities	amputation 4 extremit.	"recovery"	-	-
5-3/4-'68 La Plata, Argentina	misplaced 137Cs source found and kept in pockets	1	120 rad, mixed	uniform	asymptomatic	-	-	-	-
		1	300 - 400,000 rad γ, 3000 - 5000 rad γ, 2000 rad γ	skin vessels (upper legs) gonads	radiodermatitis (all stages) and deep necrosis	symptomatic; skin grafting (failed); amputation both legs	"recovery"	-	no gastrointestinal symptoms in spite of high dose to the abdominal region (up to 2000 rad γ)

1/ Mixed radiation consists of various types of radiation with different LET values such as neutron and gamma rays

TABLE III (continued)

PRINCIPAL RADIATION ACCIDENTS (1945 - 1975); SCHEMATIC LISTING OF EVENTS AND CONSEQUENCES

DESCRIPTION OF ACCIDENTS				RADIATION CONDITIONS		CLINICAL FINDINGS				remarks
date	location	probable cause of accident	individuals exposed and/or injured	radiation quality and dose (estimates)	dose distribution	signs and symptoms	therapy if any	clinical course	probable cause of death (if fatal)	
8-28-'68	Chicago, USA	accidental overdose of 198Au given intravenously	1	400 - 500 rad β and γ / 7000-8000 rad β and γ	bone marrow / liver	hematological syndrome	symptomatic; strict isolation	death on day 69	cerebral hemorrhage	-
9-20-'69	Glasgow, U.K.	probably misplaced 192Ir iridium source	1	20.000 rad γ / 2.000 rad γ / 1.500 rad γ	left chest / heart muscle / left hand	local ulcerations and necrosis lesion pericardium	surgical	recovery	-	-
2-4-'71	Oak Ridge, Tennessee, USA	exposure to 60Co irradiator	1	260 rad γ / 1.200 rad γ	uniform / local on hand	CNS, gastrointestinal and hematological symptoms	symptomatic	recovery with in 6 months after severe bone marrow depression	-	-
6-13-'74	Parsippany, New Jersey, USA	exposure to 60Co source	1	600 rad γ	uniform ? / bone marrow	CNS, gastrointestinal and bone marrow syndromes	conservative; isolation and decontamination	recovery after 45 days	-	-
May '75	Italy	exposure to 60Co irradiator	1	1200 rad γ / 1000 rad γ	uniform ? head / total body	CNS, gastrointestinal and hematological cal syndromes	unknown	death on day 13	gastrointestinal syndrome	-
11-20-'75	Gundremmingen, Munich, Germany	exposure to radioactive steam	2	no details given		unknown	unknown	time of death not specified	unknown	-

The main symptoms observed within the first few days after high[a]
radiation doses can be classified in a number of ways. Some authors have
introduced the concept of a "prodromal syndrome" (23) and divide its symptoms into two major groups: neuromuscular and gastrointestinal. Neuromuscular symptoms in man include: fatigue, apathy, fever, headache, hypotension,
and shock. Gastrointestinal symptoms are mainly anorexia, nausea, vomiting,
diarrhea, dehydration, and weight loss. The two categories of symptoms
often occur simultaneously, particularly at lethal dose levels which do not
lead to death within one or two days.

In this review, we do not use the expression "prodromal syndrome", but
prefer to adhere to a slightly different classification of syndromes. It is
based primarily on survival times of animals given potentially lethal and
supralethal radiation doses. Fig. 2 shows that, in mice and monkeys, so-
called cerebral death occurs within the first few days and can probably be
distinguished from intestinal death occurring between days 3 and 8 after
irradiation (14). Similar observations have since been reported for several

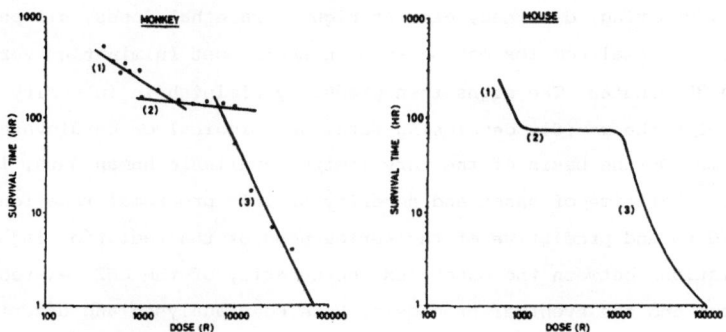

Fig. 2   Survival time following lethal whole body exposure in monkeys and mice
showing the three radiation syndromes: (1) Region of bone marrow syndrome,
(2) Plateau of intestinal syndrome, (3) Region of cerebral syndrome.
Graphs are based on data from Quastler et al., 1951 (151), Cronkite, 1951
(152) and Rajewski et al., 1953 (153) for the mouse and from Pickering et
al., 1959 (154) for the monkey. Adapted from a figure which appeared in
ref. 14 (page 29).

----

[a] potentially lethal and supralethal doses, see Table I.

other mammalian species (58). Consequently, we shall discuss these two syndromes as separate entities, fully realizing that the distinction is somewhat arbitrary and that it may be sometimes difficult to decide whether death of an individual is due to the cerebral, the intestinal, or to both syndromes simultaneously.

- ## The cerebral syndrome

This is the earliest and most fulminant type of radiation injury[a]. Time of onset, clinical course, and survival time of the individual again obviously depend on the dose and characteristics of the radiation received. After doses exceeding several thousand rad, animals and man (according to the limited human data available) develop symptoms characteristic of damage to the central nervous system or CNS (table I and figure 3). Depending on the radiation dose and characteristics, death follows within hours or maximally a few days following exposure. If the head is shielded, death can be delayed and may then be due to cardiovascular symptoms or predominantly to intestinal damage.

For man, a number of very early or prodromal symptoms have been described in detail (23). They include headache, fever, hypotension, nausea, vomiting, diarrhea, etc. At high supralethal doses, all phases of this prodomal complex can be seen in their most fulminating version within 30 minutes. The signs then gradually diminish in intensity and merge with the rapidly developing fatal neurological or cardiovascular symptoms. On the basis of the very limited available human data, it is assumed that time of onset and severity of this prodromal reaction is related to and predictive of the seriousness of the radiation injury. Associations between the onset and the severity of the CNS-related symptoms and the eventual prognosis, have been analysed and described in detail (23). There is no effective therapy for this kind of severe radiation injury.

----

[a] The more general term "radiation sickness" is purposely avoided since it has been used, without proper discrimination, for any and all types of early radiation effects.

18

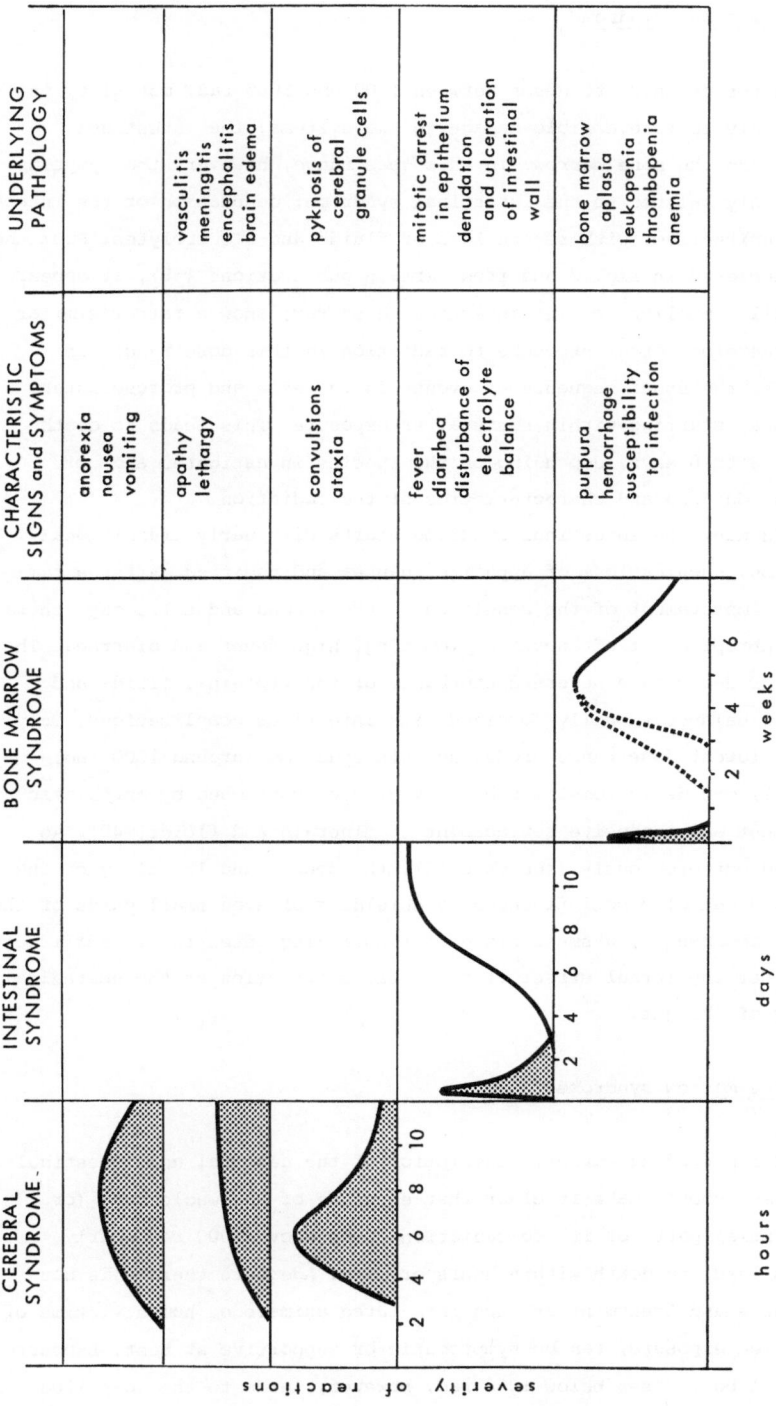

Fig. 3   Salient features of the cerebral, intestinal and bone marrow syndromes after acute radiation injury in man.
For details regarding the approximate doses of total body radiation causing these syndromes, see table I.
Stippled lines in the diagram of the bone marrow syndrome indicate that onset and time course of the syndrome are dose-dependent.
Adapted from: A.C. Upton, "Radiation injury: effects, principles and perspectives" (Chicago University Press, 1969).

The intestinal syndrome

After exposure to doses between 1000 and 5000 rad, mortality is due mainly to irreversible damage to two systems: the intestinal mucosa and the bone marrow. In this dose range, however, the symptoms are mainly related to the intestinal syndrome: denudation of the intestinal epithelium, with severe loss of fluids and electrolytes. From the data depicted in fig. 2 and from certain publications (58), it appears that all mammalian species investigated so far, show a rather similar symptomatology after exposure to radiation in this dose range. In animals, the usual sequence of events is anorexia and profuse watery diarrhea, starting within hours after exposure. This leads to death within 3 to 8 days, depending on the species investigated and, of course, on dose and characteristics of the radiation.

In man, the intestinal syndrome starts with early transitional symptoms, such as loss of appetite, nausea and vomiting. After a temporary improvement of the condition on the second and third day, there is an abrupt onset of anorexia, vomiting, high fever and diarrhea. The cause of death is a severe disturbance of the protein-, fluid- and mineral balance, usually combined with infectious complications. Only in the lowest dose range producing this syndrome (around 1000 rad; Table I) can death sometimes be prevented or postponed by antibiotic treatment and intensive replacement of minerals and fluids (49). As pointed out previously (see page 10), the course and lethality of the syndrome can also be influenced by shielding of even small parts of the ileum. Apparently, a small piece of functioning intestine is sufficient to offset the lethal effect of the total destruction of the epithelial lining of the gut.

The bone marrow syndrome

The preceding cursory description of the cerebral and intestinal syndromes should make it clear that exposure of the whole body (or substantial parts of it) to radiation doses above 1000 rad nearly always leads to death within hours or days. Adequate therapy is not available and treatment of such irradiated animals or human victims of radiation exposure, can be symptomatic or supportive at best. Exposure to total body doses below 1000 rad, however, leads to the so-called

20

bone marrow or hemopoietic syndrome which (depending on dose and quality of radiation) is also lethal, but often amenable to effective therapy. As briefly outlined in the introduction, it is this type of early radiation injury which demands our greatest attention because major advances have been made in the past decade regarding the treatment of this syndrome in man and animals. In part 4 of this report, an exposition of the current concepts of treatment of the bone marrow syndrome will be given. In this section we shall review its causative factors and symptomatology as was done for the cerebral and intestinal syndromes in the preceding paragraphs.

Animals exposed to radiation in the potentially lethal dose range (see table I) may die from failure of hemopoiesis. As already indicated, cells of the rapidly proliferating hemopoietic system (including the lymphopoietic tissue) are highly radiosensitive. After doses between about 500 and 1000 rad TBR, a rapid and serious destruction of the hemopoietic tissue occurs (14). The proliferative capacity of the hemopoietic stem cells is strongly inhibited which results in depletion of the various cellular elements in the peripheral blood. In man and animals alike, there is a disappearance of peripheral lymphocytes within 24 hours[a], of granulocytes within a few days, of platelets after about 10 days; severe anemia (due to hemorrhages caused by thrombopenia) develops within a few weeks. The time course of these events is obviously dose-dependent; fig. 4 which is based on data provided by the NRC report of '67 (23) depicts the time course and dose-dependence of those events for man. Similar data have been reported by Jammet et al. (59) and others (2). It should be clear that the very early changes observed in the peripheral blood counts of lymphocytes and platelets (and the pattern of their restoration) can be useful "monitors" to estimate the received dose and its distribution in human radiation accidents (23). Naturally, the time course, morbidity, and mortality due to the bone marrow syndrome also depend on dose, dose rate, quality (LET) and other characteristics of the radiation received.

----

[a] Unlike most other cell types, lymphocytes disintegrate within hours after irradiation, independent of mitotic events (so-called interphase death) (14).

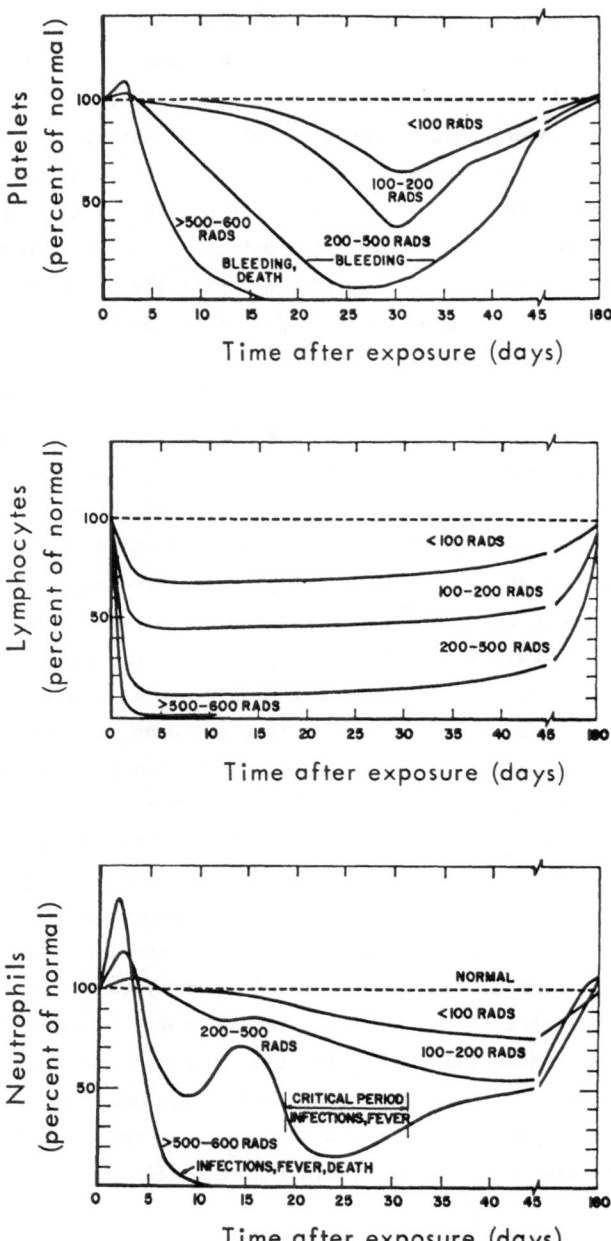

Fig. 4   Smoothed average time course of changes in lymphocyte-, neutrophil- and platelet counts in human cases from accidental radiation exposure as a function of dose.
Adapted from a figure which appeared in ref. 23 (page 95).

Unless granulocyte and platelet counts recover spontaneously (or through therapeutic measures), severe leukopenia with decreased resistance to infection (bacteremia and sepsis) and severe anemia (hemorrhages), will occur within weeks. Whether or not an individual survives a particular dose of TBR (without therapy) depends to some extent on the species, on individual resistance, and on the presence of pathogenic bacteria, fungi or viruses (pseudomonas bacteria are notorious (60)).

Dose response curves which provide the LD_{50} (the dose at which 50 % of the animals die after TBR) are available for several species and for many types and qualities of radiation (61). In general, the LD_{50} for "conventional" high intensity radiation is rather similar for most mammalian species, particularly if the many variables of experimental conditions in different laboratories are taken into account. Nevertheless, a few seemingly significant differences have been recorded. Small animals such as rodents and rabbits display a somewhat higher LD_{50} (between 500 and 800 rad, depending on radiation quality, etc.), than larger animals such as dogs, monkeys and hoofed animals (250 - 500 rad) (61). The LD_{50} for man can obviously not be "determined"; extrapolation from the few radiation accidents which permit evaluation, place the LD_{50} of man in the range of that of the large animals (23).

4. Therapy of the bone marrow syndrome

EXPERIMENTAL DATA

As indicated above, radiation doses in the potentially lethal ranges usually result in the so-called bone marrow syndrome: destruction of the hemopoietic tissue which leads to disappearance of leukocytes and platelets from the peripheral blood, with ensuing infections and hemorrhages. This syndrome can be fatal, but is amenable to therapeutic measures. As schematically depicted in table I, treatment of the bone marrow syndrome can be divided into two main categories: (a) conservative therapy (isolation, antibiotics, restoration of the fluid and mineral balance, transfusions) and (b) replacement of the victim's destroyed hemopoietic tissue with transplanted viable bone marrow cells. In this review, emphasis will be on the possibilities of bone marrow transplantation, although recent methods of isolation and bacteriological decontamination will also be briefly discussed.

The feasibility of bone marrow engraftment and its therapeutic effect in irradiated animals has been thoroughly investigated. It was first shown in the early fifties that lethally irradiated mice could be protected by shielding of the spleen (62) or by intravenous injections of bone marrow (63). Several years passed before it was proved beyond doubt that the protective effect was due to recolonisation of the host's depleted marrow by donor cells, rather than to humoral factors[a] (64, 65, 66). In the following, the principal factors which play a role in the take, efficacy and complications of transplants of hemopoietic cells from one individual to another, will be discussed.

----

[a] Shielding of small parts of the hemopoietic tissue during experimental lethal TBR is also life saving; intact stem cells will migrate to and repopulate the destroyed parts of the hemopoietic tissues (14).

Factors influencing the fate of marrow grafts

If a recipient receives a transplant from a donor who is not identical for all tissue or histocompatibility antigens, the graft will be "rejected" as a consequence of an immunological reaction against the foreign tissue antigens (67-69). Thus, the fate of any graft (skin, organ, bone marrow) is primarily dependent on the degree of histocompatibility between donor and recipient. Table IV schematically depicts the degrees of histoincompatibility to be encountered in experimental transplantation and its consequences for skin, organ, and bone marrow grafts. Only the marrow grafts will be considered in some detail.

The table indicates that if there is no histocompatibility-barrier, as in autologous or isogeneic combinations, any viable graft will "take" and will not be rejected. In allogeneic or xenogeneic situations, however, the host's immunological defences have to be significantly suppressed to permit a prolonged survival of skin and organ grafts or a take of hemopoietic cells. In the latter case, lethal total body radiation is mostly used to condition the host for the acceptance of the foreign marrow. Successful engraftment and proliferation of allogeneic cells, however, is then complicated by yet another immunological reaction, namely of the graft against the host. This Graft versus Host (GvH) reaction can lead to the potentially fatal GvH disease (GvHD), to be discussed later. The most important genetic systems which control the "strong" tissue antigens and thereby exert a major influence on the take of a graft and on the severity of GvH disease will be considered, first. Subsequently, other factors relevant for marrow engraftment and its complications, will be discussed.

-   ## The major histocompatibility complex.

Mammalian species have a chromosomal region which determines the "strong" histocompatibility antigens. This "major histocompatibility complex" (MHC) has been thoroughly investigated only in a few species: H-2 of the mouse (70-72), HLA of man (73, 74), RhLA of the rhesus monkey (75) and DLA of the dog (76). Several other mammalian species have been shown to have similar complexes, but those systems have been studied less elaborately (71). Because of its overriding influence on the fate of marrow grafts, a detailed knowledge of the MHC and its gene products is considered a prerequisite for meaningful research in

TABLE IV

HISTOCOMPATIBILITY AND FATE OF TRANSPLANTS[a]

host/donor combination	graft taken from		survival of skin	survival of vascularized organs	bone marrow grafts "take"	GvH[c]
autologous	same individual		indefinite	indefinite	easy	–
isogeneic (isologous)	member of same inbred strain or monozygous twin		indefinite	indefinite	easy	–
allogeneic (homologous)	related individual of same species	identical for MHC[b]	2–3 weeks	weeks or months	comparat. easy (imm. suppr. required)	usually mild
	unrelated individual of same species	not identical for MHC / usually not identical for markers of MHC	1–2 weeks	2 or more weeks (very variable)	strong imm. suppr. required	usually severe (depending on species and other factors d)
xenogeneic (heterologous)	individual from another species	phylogenetically close	10 days	hours or days	possible (but difficult)	severe
	individual from another species	phylogenetically widely apart	a few days (if take occurs)	minutes or hours	impossible	–

a) generalizations which are broadly valid for most mammalian species
b) MHC stands for major histocompatibility complex (see text)
c) GvH stands for Graft versus Host reaction (see text)
d) see section "Factors influencing the fate of marrow grafts"

the field of bone marrow transplantation (77). Consequently, mice, dogs and rhesus monkeys are the optimal species to serve as experimental models for clinical bone marrow transplantation.

The MHC is a "cluster" of closely linked genetic systems or loci. Most information is available for two or three highly polymorphic loci defining the SD or serologically defined antigens (named A, B and C), and for one or more loci defining reactivity in mixed lymphocyte cultures (MLR). The genetic system with an overriding influence on MLR has been called the D-locus; lymphocytes from individuals which share the D-locus antigens will not (or hardly) stimulate each other in mixed cultures. The D-locus determinants can be defined by various cellular methods and, more recently, also with antisera which identify the so-called B-cell or Ia alloantigens[a]. There are loci outside the MHC which also define histocompatibility antigens. In general, however, those other loci determine "weaker" antigens which form relatively low barriers in transplantation biology and will be disregarded for the current discussion. In man, there is also the ABO blood group system to consider when matching host and donor for bone marrow transplantation. However, numerous cases of successful marrow engraftment, in spite of incompatibility for the ABO system, have been described (17, 82, 83).

The overwhelming influence of matching for the gene products of the MHC is most easily demonstrated when transplants are exchanged between related individuals. Table IV indicates that in sibling combinations, identity for the MHC means prolonged survival of skin and organ grafts, easier takes of bone marrow and less severe GvH reactions. These basic rules seem to hold true for all species investigated.

When does MHC-identity occur and what does it mean? The best-known loci of the MHC (see above) are closely linked, which means that their genes and gene products are usually inherited "en bloc". These inheritable MHC units have been called haplotypes (84). The father provides haplotype a or b, and the mother c or d. Thus, there are 4 possible

----

[a] In the rhesus monkey (78) and in man (79) there is a strong association between the D-locus determinants and the so-called B-cell or Ia-like alloantigens. The latter are controlled by a separate locus, called Ia_1 in the rhesus monkey. Those Ia_1 antigens are probably the primates' equivalent of the murine Ia or immune-region associated antigens (80). For details see the very elaborate specialistic literature regarding those subjects (74, 81).

types of offspring regarding the MHC: ac, ad, bc, and bd. Consequently, 25 % of all siblings will be MHC-identical. Inheritance of the various haplotypes can be demonstrated by serological and cellular methods. Identical sibs have the same serologically defined antigens and are MLR negative because they share the D-locus determinants of both parental haplotypes. Recapitulating: parents and offspring share one MHC haplotype, siblings share 0, one or two MHC haplotypes. Those sharing both haplotypes are called genotypically identical; they are the allogeneic host/donor combinations with optimal results in organ and bone marrow transplantation (table IV).

In unrelated individuals of an outbred species, matching for MHC products is not so easy. In view of the extremely high polymorphism of several of the mentioned loci of the MHC (multiple alternative genes for each locus), it is difficult to find individuals who share all SD antigens and even more difficult to find combinations who share the SD antigens, the Ia antigens as well as the major D-locus determinants[a]. In spite of the many possible antigen combinations, pairs of phenotypically identical unrelated individuals can be found because of the rather high frequency of some of the antigens and because certain antigen combinations occur more frequently than would be expected by chance. This phenomenon (called linkage disequilibrium) has been observed in man, monkeys and dogs and facilitates host/donor matching in unrelated individuals (84).

In practice, matching for SD antigens is relatively simple. With an adequate battery of antisera, one can determine an individual's SD antigens and with the aid of computers (85), individuals with identical SD antigens can be traced. Matching for D-locus determinants is more difficult. Until recently, D-locus identity could only be determined by the cumbersome mixed lymphocyte culture technique (86). A few years ago, however, it was found that defining D-locus determinants may be possible also by more direct serological and cellular methods (74, 87,

----

[a] Unrelated individuals who share all the currently known identifiable MHC antigens ("phenotypic identity") need not be identical for all other determinants controlled by the MHC. In contrast, genotypically identical siblings are identical for all gene products of the MHC, provided that no "crossing-over" has taken place (84). Thus, optimally matched unrelated host/donor combinations are likely to share fewer MHC genes (and their products) than genotypically identical siblings.

88). To what extent matching unrelated individuals for the currently known SD antigens prolongs the survival of allogeneic skin and organ grafts is still a matter of controversy (89). Recent experimental work in unrelated rhesus monkeys has shown that D-locus compatibility prolongs kidney allograft survival very significantly while simple SD matching does not (90). The possible influence of matching for SD- or D-locus determinants on the fate of marrow grafts will be discussed on pages 36 and 37.

The major histocompatibility complex contains numerous other genetic systems which might influence the fate of bone marrow grafts. There are genes controlling immune responses (Ir genes (91)), genes which control "allogeneic resistance" (92), and various other MHC-linked loci. Besides there are numerous loci outside the major histocompatibility complex which may exert a noticeable influence on graft survival. However, the gene products of all those loci are still difficult to identify in most species and their significance regarding the fate of bone marrow grafts are not yet known. Therefore, they will not be further considered in the current discussions.

- Other factors influencing marrow engraftment.

As shown in table IV and briefly discussed before, the degree of histocompatibility determines to a large extent also the feasibility of marrow engraftment. A "low" histocompatibility barrier, as in MHC-identical sib combinations, facilitates engraftment, a "high" barrier makes a take of a marrow graft more difficult. In the unrelated allogeneic situation, the barrier is variable and its "height" is primarily determined by the degree of compatibility for gene products of the MHC (see above). It has also been pointed out, that in all host/donor combinations (except the isogeneic), the host has to be effectively conditioned or immuno-suppressed in order to permit the take of a foreign cellular graft. Lethal total body radiation is the method of conditioning most commonly used in experimental marrow transplantation (14) but other methods to suppress host immune reactivity are also being employed (e.g. chemotherapeutic agents, antilymphocyte serum). Sometimes the degree of immunosuppression is insufficient to permit a permanent take of a marrow graft. After sublethal radiation doses, for instance, the proliferating donor-type cells can be gradually replaced by the host's own recovering hemopoietic tissue (14). In certain mouse strain combinations, such temporary marrow grafts after sublethal radiation doses showed a deleterious effect on the host, the so-called midlethal dose or MLD-effect (93). However, this phenomenon has not been documented for other species (14, 94) and is therefore not considered an argument against bone marrow grafting after radiation accidents where individuals may have received sublethal doses.

Beside histocompatibility and the degree of immunosuppression, there are a few other factors influencing the take of a marrow graft. They include:

- the number of bone marrow cells injected. As a generalization, it can be said that the number of autologous or isogeneic bone marrow cells required for a functional take is approximately similar for all mammalian species ($3 - 5 \times 10^{7}$ cells/kg). The number of allogeneic cells required, is about 10 times higher, for most species (95). Estimates of the number of cells/kg body weight for a few species are presented in table V. For allogeneic combinations "within" a particular species, the required cell number will obviously depend on the degree of histocompatibility between donor and host.

- the route and time of injection. Intravenous application has been shown to be most efficient, requiring the lowest number of cells for effective engraftment (96). In most species, injecting the marrow within 24 hours after TBR is optimal but a beneficial effect of marrow transplantation has been observed after intervals of up to a week particularly if supportive treatment is given in the period between exposure and grafting (14).

- presensitization of the host. In allogeneic or xenogeneic combinations, immunization of the host to histocompatibility antigens carried by the bone marrow donor (e.g. by blood transfusions prior to bone marrow grafting) can jeopardize the take of a graft (97, 18).

30

TABLE V

THE NUMBER OF CELLS REQUIRED FOR A BONE MARROW GRAFT
IN DIFFERENT SPECIES

| | body weight (kg) | nucleated cells per kg body weight | | |
		isogeneic or autologous	allogeneic unmatched	proportion allog./isog.
Mouse	0.02	5×10^6	4×10^8	80
Rat	0.2	5×10^7	5×10^8	10
Guinea-pig	0.6	5×10^7	5×10^8	10
Rabbit	2.5		1×10^8	
Monkey	3	4×10^7	3×10^8	8
Dog	6	5×10^7	8×10^8	16
Calf	50	3×10^7	$>8 \times 10^8$	>25

The figures in this table represent the numbers of isogeneic, autologous and allogeneic bone marrow cells required to provide 100 per cent thirty-day survival or maximum achievable protection following lethal whole body irradiation in various species. For the monkey the criterion in case of allogeneic bone marrow, was not 30-day survival but a "take".
Adapted from a table which appeared in ref. 95 (page 319).

The Graft versus Host (GvH) reaction.

Table IV indicates that autologous or isogeneic bone marrow grafts are most easily accepted and do not lead to immunological complications. However, the availability of an isogeneic bone marrow donor (identical twin) is extremely rare in the clinical situation. Therefore, research in this area has centered on the transplantation of allogeneic bone marrow, also in outbred species such as dogs and monkeys[a]. The following section summarizes the available information.

----

[a] Several Euratom contractees are active in this field of research: G. Mullins of Dublin (contract 191-76-9 BIOEIR) and B. Dupont (217-76-1 BIOD) are involved in matching unrelated individuals for clinical bone marrow transplantation; Grosse-Wilde of Thierfelder's group in Munich (217-76-1 BIOD) does similar work in dogs, Balner and van Bekkum at the REPGO Institutes, Rijswijk (198-76-1 BION), for rhesus monkeys.

31

- Cause and pathology of GvHD.

If certain conditions are fulfilled (pages 29 and 30), allogeneic bone marrow cells will settle in the appropriate organs of the lethally irradiated individual and start proliferating. If the graft is effective, early death from infections and hemorrhages can be prevented and the animal continues to live as a cellular "chimaera"[a] (14). However, a bone marrow suspension also contains a proportion of immunocompetent lymphoid cells. These recognize the new environment as foreign and are able to mount an immunological reaction against the host, the GvH reaction. Decades of intensive research have greatly increased our understanding of the pathogenesis of the ensuing GvH disease (GvHD); yet certain aspects of this immunological complication remain to be elucidated. For unknown reasons the prime targets of the sensitized donor lymphocytes are the host's epithelial cells of skin, gastrointestinal tract and liver (98). GvH reactions probably also interfere with the restoration of the host's immune reactivity, which leads to increased susceptibility to infections in radiation chimaeras. A clear-cut distinction between the illness caused by the immunological assault on the host's target organs and the consequences of the deficient immune system, is sometimes difficult to make. In cases of fatal GvHD, the cause of death can be the former, the latter, or both.

- Patterns of GVH disease.

There are two main types of GvHD in the unmatched, allogeneic situation: (1) the delayed or rodent type, which starts a few weeks after engraftment and can lead to severe morbidity and/or mortality, mostly between day 30 and 60 after grafting. And (2) the acute or primate type which virtually always leads to very severe symptoms and death within a few weeks after grafting.

What determines the type of GvH disease? The number of mature lymphoid cells in the inoculum undoubtedly plays an important role. Fig. 5 shows that the monkey-type acute GvHD can be mimicked in mice by injecting spleen cell suspensions with a high proportion of lymphoid

----

[a] "Chimaerism" can be proved by demonstrating donor-type markers on various cell types or serum proteins (14).

cells. Primate bone marrow contains a high proportion of lymphoid cells. If this proportion is reduced (e.g. by stem cell separation; see later) the acute type of GvHD of primates is transformed into the chronic or delayed type (99). Other methods to mitigate GvHD (and thereby change its "type") will be discussed below. The type of GvHD observed in dogs is not easy to classify since data obtained in different laboratories are somewhat contradictory (100, 101, 102). Generally, the GvHD observed in unmatched host/donor combinations in dogs seems to be of the acute or primate type. However, unlike in primates, a fairly large proportion of the animals survive permanently as chimaeras (100).

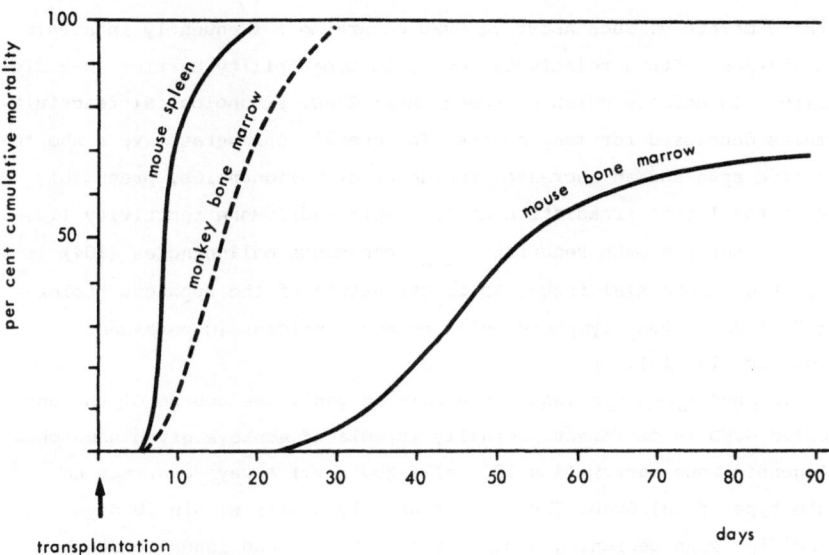

Fig. 5   Acute and delayed type of GvH disease following transplantation of allogeneic hemopoietic cells in rodents and primates conditioned with whole body irradiation. The acute reaction occurs in monkeys and man grafted with unmatched bone marrow. Since mouse bone marrow has a low content of immune competent cells, it does not induce the acute reaction, but instead the delayed type of GvH disease. The acute reaction can be induced in mice by grafting spleen cells, which contain a high proportion of immune competent cells and hemopoietic stem cells.
Adapted from a figure which appeared in ref. 121 (page 335).

33

Symptoms, histology and clinical course of GvHD.

These are basically similar for all species investigated, (including man) and are of course related to the severity of the GvHD. Symptoms and pathology can be classified according to organ involvement as presented in table VI. Detailed descriptions of the clinical course and pathology of GvHD are available for mice (14), rats (94), dogs (101), rhesus monkeys (98) and man (18, 103).

In rodents, the delayed type of GvHD usually starts with skin lesions a few weeks after grafting, often accompanied by diarrhea and a deteriorating physical condition. Severe "runting" is observed mostly during the second and third month. Depending on the strain combination (histocompatibility!), a proportion of the animals die with signs of severe GvHD, often combined with infectious lesions. However, a significant percentage does not contract the disease or recovers from it, often completely. Such abortive GvHD occurs most frequently in strain combinations with a relatively low histocompatibility barrier (H-2 disparity). In animals which overcome their GvHD, immunological reactivity remains depressed for many months. In general, chimaeras have a shortened life span and an increased incidence of malignancies, presumably due to the lethal irradiation and/or depressed immune reactivity (14, 18). Whether the GvHD reaction per se can cause malignancies (104) is still a controversial issue. So is the nature of the apparent "tolerance" of donor type lymphoid cells to host antigens in permanent chimaeras (14, 18).

In rhesus monkeys (and presumably in man), the course of the untreated GvHD is different. Lethally irradiated monkeys given unmatched allogeneic bone marrow (4 x 10^8 cells/kg, i.v.) always contract an acute type, fatal GvHD. The disease usually starts within 10 days, coinciding with beginning hemopoietic recovery, and leads to death within a week or two (median survival time about 14 days). Typical macroscopic signs of GvHD (table VI) are nearly always evident, although infectious lesions can blur the clinical picture (95).

In dogs, the clinical course of GvHD is similar, if somewhat less fulminating than in monkeys (102). However, unlike in primates, long-term surviving chimaeras have been described, also for poorly matched unrelated host/donor combinations (100).

TABLE VI

SYMPTOMATOLOGY AND PATHOLOGY OF GvH DISEASE
(generalizations for mammalian species)

rgans mainly affected	severity of the Graft versus Host Disease		
	mild	moderate	severe
SKIN symptoms	restricted erythema	- erythema - scaling - localized hairloss	- erythema - desquamation - ulceration - severe hairloss - "runted" appearance
SKIN histology	basal vacuolar degeneration and/or necrosis	- spongiosis - dyskeratosis - some epidermal necrosis	- epidermal separation and loss
NTESTINE symptoms	mild diarrhea	- moderate diarrhea - dehydration	- severe diarrhea and dehydration - disturbed mineral balance
NTESTINE histology	- isolated epithelial necrosis - dilation of glands	same lesions plus focal denudation of mucosa	diffuse mucosal denudation
LIVER symptoms	-	moderate jaundice	severe jaundice
LIVER histology	- isolated degeneration of parenchymal cells - necrosis of small bile duct epithelium	same lesions (moderate degree)	same lesions (widespread)

35

Data for humans who had received TBR in the lethal range and were treated with unmatched allogeneic bone marrow are very limited indeed (see further page 43). A few cases where additional supportive treatment was given have been described (105). They warrant the assumption that GvHD will always occur and that it will be of the acute, fulminating type. Together with monkey and dog data, this circumstance has seriously restricted the clinical application of bone marrow transplantation in the past. In the meantime, however, methods to prevent or mitigate GvHD have improved considerably. Some of the experimental approaches to decrease the incidence and severity of GvHD are described in the following section.

Methods to prevent or mitigate GvH disease

The various approaches can be divided into three major categories: (1) donor selection to achieve maximal histocompatibility, (2) improving the "quality" of the inoculum; and (3) treating the recipient before or after bone marrow grafting. Some of these methods proved highly successful in experimental work and have shown encouraging results in clinical bone marrow transplantation.

- Donor selection.

In preceding sections, it was shown that GvHD is basically the consequence of an immunological reaction of donor cells against host tissues, and that the severity and course of GvHD depend largely on the degree of histocompatibility. The all-important influence of the major histocompatibility complex was emphasized. For extrapolation to the clinical situation, the most relevant results are those obtained in experiments with dogs (106, 107) and monkeys (14), outbred species for which there is elaborate information with regard to their histocompatibility antigens. Taken as a whole, the available data reveal the following:

- related donors. Identity for the MHC, as found in genotypically identical sib combinations, significantly reduces the incidence and severity of GvHD. Nevertheless, even in such "ideal" combinations, the incidence of GvHD in dogs was about 50 % and overall

36

lethality between 10 and 25 %[a]. GvHD in these identical sib combinations is provisionally attributed to differences at "minor"
histocompatibility loci; a method to select (prospectively) siblings whose marrow will not produce GvHD, still has to be found
(107). Preliminary data for rhesus monkeys indicate that, also in
primates, the severity of GvHD is reduced when MHC identical host/
donor combinations are used (108).

-   unrelated donors. There are indications that matching for SD
    markers of the MHC reduces the incidence and severity of GvH in
    dogs (100) and in rhesus monkeys (109; Balner and van Bekkum,
    unpublished observations). However, these results need to be con-
    firmed, taking also into account other genetic markers of the MHC
    (D-locus determinants and Ia antigens, see before) and possibly
    also gene products of loci outside the MHC. Such studies are in
    progress for dogs[b] as well as rhesus monkeys[c] (110). The issue
    of selecting compatible unrelated donors is very important for
    human bone marrow transplantation since identical sibs are not
    often available in clinical situations. Some authors, working with
    inbred mouse strains, have shown that I-region or D-locus identity
    is the most important parameter to reduce GvH, as measured by the
    so-called Simonson assay (111, 112). This has led to speculations
    that D-locus identity might also be the most important parameter
    in host/donor matching for human bone marrow transplantation (17,
    113). This may well be the case; however, at the time of this
    writing, convincing data for rodents, dogs or monkeys to support
    that contention are still lacking (114).

----

[a] One laboratory reported 50 % lethality of dogs with GvHD after treatment
with marrow from DLA-identical littermates (106), the other only about
15 % (102). This difference may be due to the number of cells injected and
the kind of supportive treatment given.

[b] This subject is an integral part of the Euratom-sponsored research program
of the Gesellschaft für Strahlen- und Umweltforschung (contract 217-76-1
BIOD).

[c] Work performed under Euratom contract 198-76-1 BION at the REP-Institutes
Rijswijk.

- __Improving the quality of the inoculum.__

    Since GvHD is mainly the consequence of an immunological assault
on host tissues by immunocompetent lymphoid cells obtained in the
inoculum, numerous attempts have been made to modify the cell suspensions in such a way that the number or the immunocompetence of the
lymphoid cells is reduced while the restorative hemopoietic capacity
of the inoculum is maintained. The principal experimental avenues are:

- __other cell source__: fetal liver is a theoretical source of hemo-
    poietic cells and lymphoid precursor cells in fetal liver are
    believed to adapt more easily to allogeneic antigens (more gradual
    "tolerance" induction). Although there is some experimental evi-
    dence that the use of fetal liver cell suspensions leads to a less
    severe GvHD in rodents (115, 116), numerous technical and logistic
    drawbacks make the fetal liver an undesirable source of hemo-
    poietic cells to restore the depleted bone marrow of human beings
    (95).

- __treating the donor before marrow aspiration__: with the aim of
    reducing the number of lymphoid cells, marrow donors in animal
    experiments have been treated with various cytotoxic chemicals and
    with antilymphocyte serum (ALS). The method has been moderately
    successful in mice but not in monkeys (117). For obvious reasons,
    this approach is not particularly suitable for clinical applica-
    tion. Mathé's group has recently started a new approach to miti-
    gate GvHD in rodents: treatment of the marrow donor with high
    doses of BCG (Bacille Calmette Guérin) or Corynebacterium Parvum
    was reported to mitigate GvHD through the selective stimulation
    of donor suppressor lymphocytes (Euratom contract 220-76-1 BIOF).
    Whether this approach will be effective also in other experi-
    mental animals or in man, remains to be shown.

- __in vitro treatment of cell suspensions before transplantation__:
    numerous methods have been used, such as storing or culturing the
    cells for certain intervals under various conditions (118), pre-
    incubation with cytotoxic drugs or ALS (119), exposure to host-
    type antigens (120), etc. Some of these methods have been mode-

rately successful in rodents, i.e., the treatment delayed or mitigated the severity of GvHD. However, the results have been disappointing when tried in larger, outbred species (114).

Yet, there is one method of in vitro treatment which has been
particularly successful in animals as well as in man, namely the
separation of hemopoietic stem cells. Bone marrow and other
sources of hemopoietic cells such as the spleen contain omnipotent
stem cells as well as more differentiated elements of the ery-
throid, myeloid and lymphoid lines[a]. Numerous methods have been
devised to eliminate the more mature lymphoid elements, thus
increasing the proportion of stem cells in the suspension (121).
The method using a discontinuous albumin gradient for separation
(122) has been most thoroughly investigated with regard to the in
vivo hemopoietic capacity of the "purified" suspension. By greatly
increasing the proportion of stem cells (up to 100 fold!), a much
smaller cellular inoculum could be used to restore lethally irradiated mice and monkeys. Most importantly, GvHD was significantly
delayed or its severity reduced. In monkeys, the hyperacute GvHD
could be transformed into the delayed type which is more amenable
to supportive treatment, etc. Moreover, in vitro methods have now
become available to estimate the number of stem cells contained in
a purified suspension (123). Such stem-cell-enriched suspensions
will retain their restorative hemopoietic potential also after
freezing and storage at -196° C (124). The procedure is a major
step forward since it is capable of mitigating GvHD in the monkey
model under the worst conditions (unrelated, unmatched host/donor
combinations). The method has already been shown to be effective
also in a limited number of clinical cases (125). It should be
mentioned though, that the reduced proportion of lymphoid cells
administered can, theoretically, lead to an even slower recovery
of a chimaera's immune system which might further increase its
susceptibility to infections (126).

----

[a] Under the auspices of the Biology Division of the Commission of the European Community, Fliedner's team at Ulm University (Euratom contract
222-76-1 BIOD) is studying the characteristics and applicability of hemopoietic stem cells from peripheral blood for replacement therapy.

- <u>Treatment of the recipient before or after engraftment.</u>

  - <u>immunosuppressive treatment before grafting</u>: the aim of this
    method is, once again, reducing the proportion or the reactivity
    of the immunocompetent lymphoid cells. Various immunosuppressive
    treatments have been given in addition to (or instead of) irra-
    diation to improve conditioning[a] of the recipients for graft-
    acceptance and hopefully mitigate GvHD. In rodents as well as in
    larger animals, the administration of various immunosuppressive
    agents prior to bone marrow grafting has reduced the morbidity and
    lethality of GvHD to some degree (117). In monkeys, pretreatment
    with ALS was the most successful approach: ALS given 1 or 2 days
    before a bone marrow graft delayed and reduced GvHD and led to
    significantly prolonged survival times (127). The method is now
    also recommended for human bone marrow transplantation, particu-
    larly if an unrelated donor has to be used (see later). In the
    mouse model, a new approach to mitigate GvHD has been developed
    by Thierfelder's group in Munich; sensitization of prospective
    marrow recipients against specific T-cell antigens of the donor
    has been reported to reduce the severity of GvH reactions (128,
    Euratom contract 217-76-1 BIOD).

  - <u>immunosuppressive treatment after grafting</u>: since GvHD is prima-
    rily the consequence of an immunological reaction against "self",
    immunosuppressive treatment of the host (as applied in human auto-
    immune diseases) has been considered. Numerous immunosuppressive
    agents and a vast variety of treatment schedules have been tried.
    In general, starting the treatment <u>before</u> significant signs of
    GvHD are apparent, has been more successful than attempts to
    reverse the course of GvHD once it is established. Methotrexate
    (MTX), cyclophosphamide (CY) and ALS were among the optimal
    agents. In primates and dogs, ALS was again most effective,
    possibly because it acts somewhat selectively on T or thymus-
    dependent lymphocytes, the presumed killer cells in GvH reactions.

----

[a] In the context of this review, "conditioning" is, by definition, total
body irradiation so that other methods to obtain or improve graft-
acceptance need not be discussed in detail.

40

There is another "immunosuppressive" method which should be briefly mentioned: the application of so-called enhancing sera. In rodent experiments, it has been shown that alloantisera directed against recipient antigens sometimes reduce the severity of GvH (129). This was attributed to an "enhancing" or blocking effect of those antibodies, presumably protecting the most vulnerable host tissues against donor lymphocyte reactivity. However, Marquet and collaborators have failed to demonstrate a beneficial effect on GvHD in rats, using alloantisera which had an impressive enhancing (i.e. prolonging) effect on the survival of organ grafts in the same rat strain combination (130). In spite of these controversies regarding the efficacy of the enhancing sera in mitigating GvH reactions, the method has already been applied in clinical bone marrow transplantation, however, without success (130). It would seem that much more experimental work and a better understanding of the mechanism of enhancement is required before clinical application can be recommended.

- supportive treatment and other protective measures.

Hemorrhages: in the first 10 days after irradiation, the number of platelets may fall to a dangerous level ($<$ 20,000). Even if an effective bone marrow graft is obtained, the recovery of platelet counts may take too long to protect the animal against hemorrhages in the critical first 10 days. Transfusions of optimally matched platelets may be required to bridge this period. Such platelet suspensions should be irradiated to avoid additional GvH reactivity, caused by lymphocytes possibly contained in the suspensions.

A *disturbed fluid and mineral balance* may require adequate supportive treatment (infusions, minerals). The symptoms may be attributable to early intestinal damage caused by the irradiation or by the described GvH reaction which can lead to profuse diarrhea already in the early stages (see before).

Prevention or treatment of infectious complications is extremely important. Germfree mice or mice completely "decontaminated" (made pathogen-free by antibiotic treatment) do not die from GvHD! Thus, decontamination and isolation starting before irradiation and grafting seems a sensible preventive procedure. In this respect, results obtained with lethally irradiated monkeys given unmatched marrow are encouraging, though not yet conclusive (131). Isolation, bacteriological monitoring, and administration of irradiated, MHC-matched granulocyte suspensions may be beneficial for long-lived chimaeras since such animals remain extremely susceptible to pathogenic organisms (particularly viruses). Unfortunately, a large proportion of long-lived dog chimaeras and virtually all monkey chimaeras eventually succumb to viral infections, in spite of proper isolation, observation, and supportive treatment.

Recapitulating, it appears that the currently available measures which are aimed at reducing the number or the activity of donor-type immunocompetent cells, will indeed mitigate GvHD and prolong a chimaera's life span. However, recovery of the immune system is slow and special preventive and/or therapeutic measures are required to guard against infection, the most serious late complication of GvHD.

Bone marrow transplantation after accidental radiation.

There are only a few documented cases of human bone marrow transplantation after accidental lethal irradiation (Table III). In one single case,
an identical twin was available as marrow donor. In such a host/donor combination, which is comparable to isogeneic transplantation in animals, the
conditions for a take are optimal and immunological complications are not
anticipated. According to the scarce documentation of the case, engraftment
was indeed uneventful and the transplant was considered life-saving (132).

The remaining cases are the victims of the Vinča accident of 1958, in
which 5 men and 1 woman received potentially lethal radiation doses. Eventually, five of them were treated with marrow grafts from unrelated, allogeneic donors. Their case histories have been well documented (59, 133,
134) and can be summarized as follows. The various dose estimates (tables
III and VII) and the early clinical course, permitted the conclusion that
at least 5 of the 6 patients had been exposed to doses exceeding the LD_{75}.

TABLE VII

ESTIMATED NEUTRON AND GAMMA DOSES RECEIVED BY PERSONS
INVOLVED IN THE "VINCA ACCIDENT" OF 1958

patient	Jammet (73)		Hurst and Ritchie (67)		Auxier (3)		
	neutron (rem)	gamma (rem)	neutron (rem)	gamma (rem)	charged particle dose (rad)	H (n,γ)D gamma dose (rad) [a]	total radiation dose (rad)
V	210	630	320	320	89	133	214
M	214	642	290	290	87	130	209
G	230	690	300	300	90	135	189
D	256	768	250	250	91	136	192
H	174	522	210	210	66	99	158
B	102	306	175	175	45	67	95

[a] Neutron capture in hydrogen resulting in deuterons and 2.2 MeV gamma-rays.
Adapted from a table which appeared in ref. 14 (page 196).

The victims thus became candidates for marrow grafts although the risks of transplanting marrow from unrelated donors was well recognized, already at that time. After a short observation period in Belgrade, the casualties were flown to Paris and treated by a team headed by Jammet and Mathé (59). Barrier-nursing was applied and supportive treatment (antibiotics, transfusions, etc.) was given before as well as after marrow transplantation. The most heavily irradiated patient first received 4×10^9 spleen and liver cells from a human fetus which did not lead to hemopoietic recovery. His condition deteriorated, also after a bone marrow graft taken from an unrelated unmatched donor was given on day 27. The patient died a few days later, probably due to massive hemorrhages. Four other patients were given $8.5 - 14 \times 10^9$ bone marrow cells, also from unrelated donors. This was followed by gradual hemopoietic recovery. Erythrocytic chimaerism could be demonstrated until about 2 months after grafting but no signs of GvHD were observed. Two years later, the only remaining symptoms were low lymphocyte counts in all cases, and azoospermia in two patients.

It is impossible, even now, to draw firm conclusions regarding the necessity of performing those transplants, or about their contribution to the rapid hemopoietic recovery (15). However, in view of the prolonged azoospermia, it seems likely that the temporary bone marrow grafts had been life-saving in at least two cases. Furthermore, the results indicated that temporary takes of bone marrow from unmatched, unrelated donors are feasible and could be of therapeutic value in the treatment of serious radiation injury (see also section 5 of this review).

Bone marrow transplantation for other indications.

Since the time of the pioneering marrow transplants after the Vinča accident, a considerable amount of new information has been accumulated and bone marrow transplantation has become a widely accepted adjunct therapy for several other clinical indications. The experience gained in the past décade by a limited number of clinical workers has led to reasonable agreement about principles and logistics of modern bone marrow transplantation. With minor modifications, these principles are also valid for marrow transplantation after radiation accidents. For that reason, the experience and conclusions of the most active clinical teams will be briefly reviewed.

At present, the major indications for clinical bone marrow grafting are: marrow aplasia, leukemia, and combined immune deficiency diseases (CID). There are six teams of clinical workers who published the results of rather large series of patients treated with marrow grafts. They are the teams in Seattle (E.D. Thomas and R. Storb), in Paris (G. Mathé and L. Schwarzenberg), in Bethesda (R.D. Graw), in Baltimore (G. Santos), in Minnesota (R.A. Good), and in Holland (L.J. Doorn and J.J. van Rood).

In the coming section we shall briefly outline the experiences of these groups and their conclusions[a]. Emphasis will be on aspects of their work which might have bearing on the "strategy" for the treatment of radiation casualties (section 5 of this review). But first, we shall give a short account of the few documented cases of isogeneic and autologous marrow grafts. These are discussed separately, since they do not entail the immunological problems encountered in the grafting of allogeneic marrow.

- Isogeneic and autologous marrow grafts.

It is understandable that the number of documented cases of isogeneic transplants is limited, since monozygotic twin siblings are not often available as marrow donors. Nevertheless, the Seattle group (18) described 10 cases of aplasia, not due to radiation exposure, which were treated in this fashion. In 50 % of the cases successful engraftments were obtained which led to total hemopoietic recovery. A review of all cases of isogeneic transplants up to '71, led to the tentative conclusion that the minimum number of isogeneic cells required for a functional take can be estimated to be $1 - 2 \times 10^8$ cells/kg body weight (95). Thomas and collaborators (Seattle) published the largest series of leukemia patients treated with identical twin marrow[b]. The results in that series of nearly 30 cases were considered to be favorable (18).

With regard to the transplantation of preserved autologous marrow cells, data are still scarce and difficult to interpret[a]. The literature describes mostly patients with hematological malignancies, who were given autologous marrow aspirated during remissions of their disease. Frequent failures of engraftment in those cases have been attributed to poor recovery of viable stem cells after thawing the frozen cell suspensions (114). Now that reliable methods have been developed to "measure" the proportion of viable stem cells in preserved marrow (124), the actual size of the cellular inoculum can be determined more accurately and better clinical results can be expected. Optimal stem cell recovery from preserved marrow is highly relevant to the treatment of acute radiation injury in man where "banking" of autologous and/or matched allogeneic marrow may play an important role (section 5 of this review).

- Allogeneic bone marrow grafts.

In the section dealing with experimental data, it was emphasized that histocompatibility barriers are all-important for various aspects of allogeneic marrow grafting: the "take", the severity of GvHD and the subsequent fate of the chimaera (recovery of immune competence, etc.). It was also pointed out, that within the category of allogeneic host/donor combinations, genotypically identical siblings (MHC-identical) are the most favourable combination, by far. The clinical experience of the past 15 years, confirmed that conclusion: only the use of marrow from MHC-identical siblings[b] can be regarded as comparatively safe. At the time of writing, any other combination (unmatched related and well-matched unrelated) entails a great risk, even if optimal procedures to mitigate GvH disease are applied. This should explain why, in the vast majority of published cases, only MHC-identical siblings have been used as marrow donors.

----

[a] One of the Euratom contractees, P. Stryckmans of Brussels University, is currently investigating the possible inhibitory influence of granulocyte transfusions on the take and proliferation of autologous marrow transplants in man (Euratom contract 161-76-1 BIOB).

[b] Other close relatives (uncles, nephews) can also be MHC-identical but that is a very rare event.

The Seattle group provides the largest series of well-documented cases of allogeneic marrow transplants performed in a single center (18). By February '74, 37 patients with m̲a̲r̲r̲o̲w̲ ̲a̲p̲l̲a̲s̲i̲a̲ had been treated with MHC-matched sibling marrow. The majority were aplasias of unknown origin. Most patients were conditioned with Cyclophosphamide[a] (CY); nine were conditioned with TBR (^{60}Co, 1000 rad). Methotrexate (MTX) was given intermittantly after grafting to combat possible GvHD. Results were encouraging since 33/37 patients showed engraftment, proved by hemopoietic recovery and other methods. Six patients died with GvHD between day 19 and 95. Sixteen patients were alive with functioning grafts at the time of publication (1975).

In September 1976, the International Bone Marrow Transplant Registry published a detailed report on the results of treating marrow aplasia by grafting HLA-matched bone marrow; the results obtained in Seattle were compared with the pooled results obtained elsewhere. Fig. 6

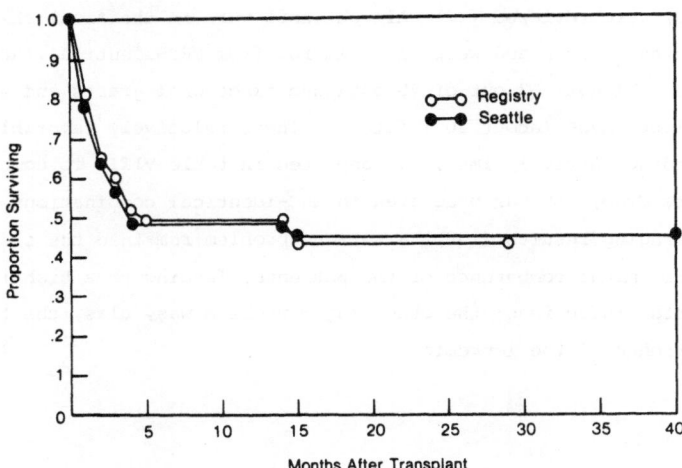

Fig. 6   Life table analysis of 75 patients with aplastic anemia who were treated with transplants of bone marrow from HLA-matched allogeneic donors.
Adapted from a figure which appeared in ref. 135 (page 1134).

---

[a] using the "Baltimore schedule"; see page 51.

demonstrates that the survival experience in the two series was
similar. The publication also revealed that the prognosis is fourfold
better if the marrow transplant is performed within 3 months of diagnosis[a), that patients $>$ 21 years had a significantly higher survival
rate than those $<$ 21 years of age. Also, survival rates were significantly higher for patients who had received 15 or fewer pre-transplant
transfusions than those who had received more than 15 transfusions
(135). In the latest publication by the Seattle group which provides
the results for 49 patients, the overall outcome was similarly
promising: 41 % of all marrow-treated patients showed long-term survival (136). A statistical analysis by members of the same team revealed
unequivocally that marrow transplantation gives significantly better
results than conventional therapy of aplasia (137).

The Seattle group also provides the largest series of leukemia
patients treated with allogeneic marrow. Seventy patients with acute
lymphatic leukemia (ALL, 36 cases) or acute myeloid leukemia (AML, 34
cases) were reviewed (18). All patients were in the final chemotherapy-
resistant stages and were given marrow from MHC-identical, ABO compatible siblings; 63 out of 70 obtained functional grafts and 46 of those
developed GvHD (about 20 % fatal!). These relatively favorable results
regarding survival times, are depicted in table VIII. To combat the
severe GvHD, ALS was used even in MHC-identical combinations and with
encouraging results (138). A serious problem remained the slow recovery
of the immune competence of the patients, leading to a high incidence
of fatal infections; the other major problem was, alas, the frequent
recurrence of the leukemia.

----

a) 55 % of patients who received bone marrow within three months after the
diagnosis of aplasia were alive at the end of 1975.

TABLE VIII

ALLOGENEIC MARROW TRANSPLANTS FOR ACUTE LEUKEMIA
USING HLA MATCHED SIBLING DONORS (SEATTLE EXPERIENCE)

	total no. cases	no. in remission >3 months	no.	median time to relapse (months)	range (months)	survival of patients now in remission (months)
acute lymphatic leukemia (ALL)	34	19	11[a]	2.5	0 - 18[b]	49, 31, 20, 19, 13, 6, 5, 4, 3
acute myeloid leukemia (AML)	36	14	4	1.5	0 - 6	29, 23, 16, 12, 7, 5, 4, 3, 3, 3

[a] Five patients were prepared with TBR only

[b] One patient relapsed at 18 months. All other patients relapsed in < 7 months

Adapted from a table which appeared in ref. 18 (page 840)

The Paris group is well known for its pionering work in the field of allogeneic marrow grafting (15). After the described Vinca-episode which proved the feasibility of allogeneic marrow grafting in man (see above), Mathé and collaborators chose the treatment of acute leukemia as their prime field of interest[a]. They added a dimension, by using the inevitable GvH reactions as adjunct therapy to combat leukemia ("GvL"). A middle way between a sufficiently effective GvL and a mild GvH was the ultimate goal! In the early sixties, conditioning of the patients was done mainly by TBR (^{60}Co, 800 rad) and the donor marrow was taken from related or unrelated individuals (often from multiple donors). It was proved that restoration of hematological function after lethal TBR was possible (17 patients) and that transitory but long remissions could be achieved in some of the patients (103). Unfortunately, all patients eventually died from GvHD, recurrent leukemia, or

----

[a] Mathé and collaborators are still active in this field, under Euratom contract 220-76-1 BIOF. The main interest remains an optimal definition of the indications for bone marrow transplantation in cases of aplasia and refractory leukemia.

both. The final conclusion had to be that GvHD was too great a hazard
if MHC-non-identical donors were used. In the past decade, the methods
of "conditioning" the patients for grafting were gradually changed.
In 38 patients (24 with aplasia, 14 with leukemia) conditioning was
done with ALS only. This approach drastically reduced the incidence of
GvHD, but takes occurred less frequently and were usually temporary and
"partial" (15).

Drawing conclusions from the Paris data is rather difficult. Only
a few of the donors were MHC-identical siblings; in many cases, multiple donors (related and unrelated) had been used. Not surprisingly
(in retrospect!), the use of marrow from MHC non-identical poorly
matched donors had led to fatal immunological complications in the
majority of cases. In spite of these inevitably disappointing early
results, Mathé and colleagues continued their programs with admirable
perseverance and can therefore be regarded as the "parents" of modern
clinical marrow transplantation.

The Bethesda group started reexamining the therapeutic potential of
allogeneic marrow transplantation in '69. They treated leukemic
patients who were refractory to chemotherapy. The main incentives were
the spectacular progress in histocompatibility testing and matching as
well as the improved possibilities of supportive care. Initially, conditioning was done with CY[a] (12 patients) and 3 patients were conditioned with TBR (950 rad, γ-rays). MTX was given regularly post-
transplant as a precaution against GvHD. The donors were MHC-identical
sibs, only. More recently, a new method of conditioning which included
CY plus 3 other chemotherapeutic agents was tried (16). This regimen
(called BACT) was given in a 4- or 6-day course prior to grafting and
was considered superior to the conventional CY-conditioning. Interestingly, the use of ABO incompatible MHC-identical sib donors led to
proper engraftment in several cases, particularly if the patient was
given the incompatible blood group substance prior to conditioning.
The use of ALS to combat incipient GvHD was considered beneficial,
also by these investigators (82).

----

[a] using the "Baltimore schedule" as described in the next paragraph.

The Baltimore group introduced a new method of conditioning in the late sixties[a]. The first 8 cases (mostly acute myelocytic leukemia or AML) included 3 or 4 patients given marrow from non-identical sibling donors. Consequently, the incidence and severity of GvHD was high. More recently, only MHC-identical sibling donors were used, some of them incompatible for the ABO blood group system. The number of cells injected was around 2×10^8 cells/kg. By 1974, the series included 8 cases of AML and 2 cases of ALL (acute myeloid and lymphatic leukemia, respectively). The results showed that engraftment was obtained in all but one case, that there may have been some anti-leukemic effect, that GvHD was present in four, but lethal in only one case. Five of the 10 patients died with interstitial pneumonitis, a "score" comparable to that of most other clinical teams. Again, incompatibility for the ABO system did not seem to affect engraftment or the severity of GvHD (83).

The Minnesota group as well as *the Dutch investigators* concentrated on the treatment of combined immune deficiency diseases (CID). The main "logistic" difference with marrow transplantation in leukemic or aplastic patients, is that conditioning of the patients (with TBR or chemotherapy) is not required, that the threshold dose of donor cells necessary to obtain a graft is lower and that prior transfusions etc. will not sensitize the patients to future donor antigens. Also the patients' immunological unresponsiveness allows a frequent repetition of marrow grafts from the same compatible donor (139).

   An impressive series of successfully treated CID cases have been published. Good et al. treated 14 infants with CID (17). In six cases, the donors were MHC identical sibs; three of these showed complete immunological recovery and are alive and well 2 - 4 years after transplantation, three died within a few weeks of intercurrent infections. Two others received marrow from an SD non-identical, MLC-negative sib; both patients are alive and well. From these two cases, the possibly premature conclusion was drawn that D-locus identity is the most important parameter in matching for marrow grafting. Most infants

----

[a] Patients are given 500 ml donor blood on day -5, then 50 mg/kg cyclophosphamide (CY) i.v. on 4 successive days. Marrow grafting is performed 24 h later and CY (7.5 mg/kg) is again given post-transplant on days 1, 3, 5, 7 and 9.

obtained multiple marrow transplants (1×10^6 to 1×10^9 cells/kg, per graft). The incidence and severity of GvHD was low in the MHC identical group, but high in the unmatched combinations.

A special feature of the "Dutch approach" is the use of hemopoietic stem cell concentrates (125, 140). Rationale and advantages of this method have been discussed on page 39. The results obtained in a series of 10 infants suffering from severe CID, who were treated with stem-cell concentrates between 1968 and 1973 have been reviewed by van Bekkum (139). It appeared that two of the three individuals who received stem cell concentrates from MHC-identical donors recovered completely (current survival 4 and 6 years). The average number of cells given (in all 10 cases) was 5×10^6/kg which is considerably lower than the average number of unfractionated marrow cells given by the other groups. It was concluded that, if stem cell concentrates are employed, the notorious acute GvHD can often be prevented even when non-matched allogeneic marrow is given (139). However, the delayed GvHD which develops, can easily lead to fatal infections so that strict isolation and, if possible, antibiotic decontamination of the patients is strongly recommended.

In the latest report from the International Bone Marrow Transplant Registry (March, 1977) the results of marrow transplantation in CID were reviewed (145). A total of 69 registered cases were considered. The overall prognosis is now regarded as very promising: of the patients treated with marrow (or marrow stem cells) from MHC-identical sibs, 63 % had been cured; however, the prognosis for those treated with non-identical marrow was rather poor. An interesting new aspect was the observation that GvHD occurred more frequently in male patients, especially when given marrow from female donors!

Recapitulating, the results obtained by six medical teams which performed the vast majority of clinical marrow transplants in the past decade, permit the following provisional conclusions:

-   bone marrow transplantation has become an established adjunct
    therapy for marrow aplasia and several types of acute leukemia
    and is the therapy of choice for the treatment of severe CID,
    provided that an MHC-identical sibling donor is available.

- autologous or isogeneic transplants (from identical twins) are
  uniformly successful if a sufficient number of viable cells is
  given. Improved techniques of cell preservation and in vitro
  techniques to monitor stem cell viability will increase the
  applicability of such therapy and facilitate the creation of
  "marrow banks" (see section 5).

- allogeneic marrow transplants from MHC non-identical donors are
  feasible if host-immunity is adequately suppressed and if the
  inoculum is sufficiently large $(2 - 4 \times 10^8$ cells/kg or an
  "equivalent" number of gradient-separated stem cells). However,
  the risk of severe GvHD and subsequent fatal infections is unduly
  high, even if optimal methods to mitigate GvHD are applied.
  Altered methods of host-conditioning (CY or CY plus ALS, instead
  of TBR) reduce the severity of GvHD but may lead to incomplete
  engraftment and do not significantly reduce the risk of late,
  fatal infections. The use of stem cell concentrates combined with
  decontamination and isolation of the patient may reduce those
  risks to an acceptable level.

- allogeneic marrow transplants from MHC-identical donors have been
  shown to be relatively "safe". If conditioning is adequate, $2 - 4$
  $\times 10^8$ cells/kg (or 5×10^6 gradient-separated stem cells per kg)
  usually lead to a functional take. In about 50 % of such cases,
  GvHD will occur and in half of these cases it can be fatal. As
  yet, no methods are available to determine, beforehand, whether
  or not GvHD will occur. In selecting compatible sibling donors
  there are some indications (but no proof) that incompatibility
  for the ABO blood group system can be disregarded and, concerning
  the major histocompatibility complex, that identity for D-locus
  determinants may be more important than SD identity.

- antilymphocyte serum is, at present, the optimal immunosuppressant
  to reduce the incidence and severity of GvHD prior to its occurrence. It may also be useful in treating GvHD, once it has
  appeared.

53

- The slow restoration of the immune capacity of human chimaeras remains a major problem, also if marrow from MHC-identical donors has been used. Prolonged isolation is recommended and, if possible, antibiotic decontamination of the patients prior to grafting should be considered.

5. Strategy for the treatment of severe radiation injury in man

The guidelines given in this section schematically describe the necessary facilities and principal measures to be taken in the case of radiation accidents, particularly those which may ultimately require bone marrow transplantation. Thus, we shall attempt to delineate a strategy for the treatment of individuals after serious partial or total body exposure to external radiation sources. The equally important issue of how to treat individuals after internal or external contamination with radioactive material is dealt with in a very cursory fashion only, since bone marrow transplantation will rarely be required after such contamination. There is a large body of literature dealing with that specific subject (142, 143).

GENERAL PRINCIPLES

Most health authorities of nations with an advanced nuclear potential (power plants, production of radioisotopes, etc.) have established certain guidelines for the handling of victims of radiation accidents. Some of those "strategies" were reviewed at a recent symposium in Vienna (144, 145, 146, 147). Although national guidelines may differ in detail, the general principles are rather similar for most countries and can be broadly summarized as follows:

- The handling of accidents should be done in a regional fashion, by which smaller nations might share the required specialized medical facility (see below) and thus represent a single "region".

- The regions should function at three operational levels, namely (1) the site of the accident, (2) a support hospital in the vicinity, equipped with radiation emergency areas for decontamination, etc. and (3) a regional medical center which has expertise in the most modern and sophisticated diagnostic and therapeutic procedures for definitive medical care.

- Each diagnostic and/or therapeutic echelon should nominate one individual (preferably a physician trained in radiation medicine) who is
available on a 24-hr basis and is responsible for the smooth coordi-
nation of all required therapeutic activities.

Most national programs also emphasize the importance of regular
training courses to update treatment methods, repeated inventory of emergency equipment and supplies and frequent exercises involving simulated
accidents to check the state of preparedness. Some health authorities have
issued brochures which describe the requirements for the facilities for
immediate "on site" treatment. It is suggested that, particularly in cases
where external or internal contamination has taken place, emergency decontamination and surgical treatment should be carried out at the site of the
accident; this should otherwise be done at the nearby support hospital
where special decontamination areas and facilities should be available. It
is generally recommended that the taking of biosamples[a] start as early as
possible and be continued at regular intervals.

We shall now offer suggestions for the handling of accidents in which
potentially life-threatening external radiation has taken place. This includes a brief description of the prototype of a specialized regional medical center, the steps to be taken if a bone marrow transplant is considered,
the "logistics" of such a transplant if required and, finally, speculations
about future bone marrow banks.

INITIAL STEPS AT THE VARIOUS MEDICAL FACILITIES

In peacetime, accidental radiation exposure is most likely to occur
at the site of nuclear research or industry. Here, the main tasks will be
providing optimal first aid to keep the patient alive while removing him
from the radiation area, applying external and/or internal decontamination
(if required), taking the first bioassay samples and preparing the patient
for transport to the nearby support hospital. Requirements for emergency

----

[a] These include saliva, urine, feces, blood and bone marrow. Regular sample
taking is essential for the subsequent evaluation of the severity of an
accident.

treatment facilities at the location of nuclear research or industry have been lucidly described by Linneman and Mettler (147). The same authors have stressed the importance of optimal lines of communication among the individuals in charge at the site of the accident and those at the support hospital and the specialized regional center.

The support hospital, located in the immediate neighbourhood, should take care of further emergency treatment (mostly surgical) and start the evaluation of the victim's "radiation status". The mentioned contact between the responsible staff at this hospital, the experts at the plant and at the specialized regional center (see below) will provide guidelines for further treatment. The support hospital requires special provisions to permit safe treatment of potentially contaminated patients in so-called radiation emergency areas. Experience in the United States has shown that, in the majority of cases, the complete handling of accidents will take place at the support hospital, not at the much larger regional centers (147).

It may take 2 or 3 days until the physical and radiation status of the patient is sufficiently clear to determine the further course of the treatment. If results of a reconstruction of the accident and the victim's hematological evolution do not exclude a potentially lethal radiation exposure, the patient will have to be transferred to the regional center. At this time, the victim's relatives, especially siblings, should be requested to stand-by for possible donations of blood or bone marrow.

The Specialized Regional Center (SRC) should be a large medical complex capable of further evaluation and treatment of any type of radiation accident. One or two staff members, preferably hematologists, should act as "liaison officers" for referral of the patient(s), for maintaining contacts with the experts at the site of the accident and the local support hospital as well as for contacts with relatives. These individuals will head a "radiation medicine unit" within the SRC and require the continuous formalized support of consultants who are experts in the fields of health physics, radiobiology, radiation medicine, etc. The availability of a mobile medical emergency team at the SRC has also been recommended. Such a unit could be sent out to assist in the initial evaluation of the patient's radiation status, the appropriate cleaning-up of the area of the accident, the initial emergency treatment, etc. For the handling of severe bone marrow depression, the center needs certain facilities, which include the following:

- modern departments of medicine and surgery, with the capability of
handling not one, but numerous potential victims of serious radiation
accidents. In view of the scarcity of such accidents (which implies the
danger of long periods of idleness), radiation medicine units should be
in routine operation within the department of medicine, with the provi-
sion that space required for radiation victims could be made available
at very short notice.

- immediate access to well-equipped clinical laboratories; this includes
laboratories capable of handling any type of hematological, bacteriological or immunological problem on a 24 hour basis. The staff of the
hematological laboratory should collaborate closely with teams who are
familiar with modern techniques of cell preservation, gradient separation of cells from blood or bone marrow and the in vitro determination
of hemopoietic stem cell viability, also after preservation.

- a large isolation unit which should be operational at all times. Such
units exist in medical centers where so-called barrier nursing is
applied for tumor chemotherapy, for the treatment of immune deficiency
diseases, serious burns, etc. The aim is to protect the patient from
environmental sources of infection. If necessary, antibiotic decontamination of the patient should be performed[a].

- a laboratory for tissue typing should also be on the premises or in the
immediate vicinity and should be operative on a 24-hr basis. Its staff
should be familiar with the most advanced techniques for serological
and cellular typing and matching procedures for histocompatibility.
Tissue typing laboratories are often "affiliated" with conventional
isolation units where bone marrow transplantation can be essential for
the treatment of a variety of disorders (see section 4).

----

[a] Protocols for antibiotic decontamination can be obtained from the Gnoto-
biotic Project Group of the EORTC (European Organization for Research on
Treatment of Cancer, Institut Jules Bordet, 1 Rue Héger-Bordet, 1000
Brussels, Belgium).

After on-site emergency treatment, decontamination, sample taking and a possible observation period at the local hospital, the victim may have to be referred to the specialized regional center for possible bone marrow transplantation. The following section covers the steps to be taken under these circumstances. Such "rules" are clearly subject to frequent alterations, since immunological and hematological procedures have to be regularly adapted to the latest and most promising results obtained in experimental work[a].

a)   the initial period

   -    the patient should be placed in an isolation unit (after required emergency treatment for shock, fractures, burns, etc., has been carried out).

   -    the hematological status should be monitored at regular intervals; this includes bone marrow aspirations for smears, mitotic counts and determination of the colony forming potential.

   -    the immunological and bacteriological status should be monitored. If necessary, antibiotic decontamination should be performed.

   -    complete tissue typing of the victim as well as of all available close relatives should be performed. Siblings who are identical for the major histocompatibility complex (MHC) should be persuaded to stand-by in case a marrow transplant is required. If no MHC-identical sibling is available, attempts should be made to locate unrelated volunteer marrow donors of optimal histocompatibility (according to the latest criteria). A maximal number of other genetic markers (blood groups, enzymes, serum proteins, etc.) of the victim and the potential donor(s) should be determined to permit the subsequent demonstration of chimaerism.

----

[a] Updated information on internationally standardized methods of bone marrow transplantation is available through publications of the International Bone Marrow Registry (Mount Sinai Med. Center, Milwaukee, Wi, USA) or the chairman of its advisory committee.

-   immunosuppressants such as antilymphocyte globulin as well as
    other (contemporary) agents to prevent or combat GvHD should be
    readily available.

b)   the intermediate observation period

There are only two possible courses the clinical picture can take,
namely, improvement or deterioration.

1.   if the general condition, prodromal symptoms and daily hematolo-
     gical examinations indicate improvement, the patient is kept in
     isolation and under close observation until there is reasonable
     certainty that a marrow transplant will not be required. Until
     that time, blood transfusions from potential marrow donors should
     be avoided. If transfusions must be given, GvH reactions may occur
     and appropriate measures to mitigate such reactions should be
     taken (see section 4, pages 36 to 41). When granulocyte and
     platelet counts have stabilized at approximately normal levels
     and lymphocyte counts are not less than 50 % of normal, the
     patient can be transferred to a regular medical unit.

2.   if the general condition, prodromal symptoms and/or hematological
     examinations show deterioration, a marrow transplant should be
     considered. Whether or not it should be carried out depends
     largely on:

     -   the severity of the patient's condition: increasingly severe
         CNS, cardiovascular and gastrointestinal symptoms may be
         signs of excessive exposure (see table I); in such cases a
         marrow transplant would be futile.

     -   the availability and collaboration of a suitable donor, which
         includes (in order of preference) an MHC-identical sibling or
         an optimally matched related or unrelated volunteer donor[a].

----

[a] Obviously, the administration of autologous marrow (preserved prior to the
accident) or marrow from an identical twin would be optimal. However, since
preservation of autologous marrow is not yet practised as a precautionary
measure and the availability of an identical twin is very rare, both alternatives can be disregarded.

60

- the final outcome of a thoroughly worked out estimate of
  dose, quality and distribution of the radiation received
  (according to results of a mock-up simulation of the accident).

Once the decision to perform a transplant is taken, then certain con-
secutive steps which will be schematically outlined in the following section, can be taken. Again, such a listing may soon be obsolete in view of
the progress expected from the work of numerous teams engaged in fundamental and applied research in these areas.

c) Logistics of a marrow transplant

There are two alternative situations to be discussed: the relatively favorable one when an MHC-identical sibling is available and
willing to donate bone marrow and the rather unfavorable situation when
no MHC-identical sibling is available. As in the preceding sections,
the suggestions which follow are based on information available at the
time of writing. Both alternatives will be dealt with in a highly schematic fashion.

1. An MHC-identical sibling is available as marrow donor.

According to the literature, the i.v. administration of $2 - 4 \times 10^8$
viable bone marrow cells will usually lead to a take of the graft
(assuming, as we do here, that the exposure has been in the lethal
range). Unfortunately, the injection of crude marrow cell suspensions will lead to a rather high incidence of serious GvHD, even
in this "ideal" host/donor combination, 50 % of cases may contract
GvHD and 25 % may have a fatal outcome. The following mitigating
procedures should therefore be considered:

- the administration of methotrexate at regular intervals after
  grafting as indicated in ref. 18.

- antilymphocyte globulin (ALG), to be given daily after the
  first signs of GvHD appear. In view of the possible sensiti-
  zation to foreign proteins, the availability of ALG's prepared in two different species (e.g. rabbit-anti-human and
  horse-anti-human) is recommended.

- the use of gradient separated stem cell preparations instead
of crude marrow, if a sufficient quantity of donor marrow is
available (the average loss during stem cell separation is
about 50 %). This approach is recommended, especially if the
recipient is male and the marrow donor an MHC-identical
female (see page 52).

The decision whether (and which of) these alternatives will
be applied depends to some extent on the personal preference and
previous experience of the team leader. The first alternative
seems least hazardous and least beneficial; the second depends
largely on the quality of the available ALG. The third is probably
the most effective method to avoid lethal GvHD, but requires considerable experience with cell separation techniques (see also
section 4, pages 39 and 52).

2.   An MHC-identical sibling is not available as marrow donor.

Here, the decision of whether or not to perform a transplant is
much more difficult. The estimate of the quantity and probable
distribution of the radiation received, will be of major influence
on the decision.

- If the exposure was homogeneous and will clearly lead to
fatal intestinal and/or CNS injury ($\gg$ 1000 rad), a marrow
graft cannot be expected to be of therapeutic value.

- If the exposure was sublethal, the grafting of allogeneic
marrow can be beneficial by tiding the patient over a temporary marrow aplasia and decreasing the susceptibility to
infections. GvHD, if present, would not persist long enough
to endanger the patient's life. If the dose was substantially
below 200 rad, the graft is likely to be rejected before GvHD
can develop.

- A serious dilemma exists in cases of potentially lethal
  radiation doses (200 - 1000 rad). Here, the choice is between
  conservative therapy (and the risk of hemopoietic death) and
  a transplant of marrow, which, even if obtained from an unrelated donor who is optimally matched for histocompatibility, entails the risk of very serious GvHD.

In case of grafting, the options to reduce the likelihood of
lethal GvHD are similar to those mentioned under (1), but much
more pressing: a) the patient should receive ALG; however, in
this situation, ALG should be given shortly before transplantation as well as at the time of GvHD; b) the administration of
gradient-separated stem cell preparations instead of crude marrow
is strongly recommended. The advantage of the latter approach is
a certain delay of the GvHD and reduction of its severity. The
disadvantage is a slightly reduced chance of obtaining a "take"
and possibly a somewhat slower recovery of the host's immune
reactivity (infections!).

In patients treated with marrow from MHC non-identical
donors, the occurrence of chronic GvHD is a virtual certainty;
however, this risk has to be accepted in view of the criticality
of the situation. Consequently, there will be a prolonged period
in which the patient will be seriously ill and in which depression
of immune reactivity is a salient feature. Protection against
viral and other infections in this period is particularly important. Therefore, the patient should be treated under strict isolation and antibiotic decontamination should always be attempted.

"MARROW BANKS"

The encouraging results of clinical bone marrow transplantation and
modern cell storage techniques have led to a renewed interest in the concept of "marrow banks". The following and last section of this review repre-
sents the author's personal ideas about the desirability of establishing
such banks in the not too distant future and some of their characteristics.
At the time of writing, marrow banking is certainly not yet a realistic

63

approach. Arguments against the immediate establishment of marrow banks are:
(1) the low number of radiation accidents which have so far required marrow
transplantation; (2) the need to collect marrow from healthy donors under
full anesthesia, which entails a minimal but not negligible risk; and (3)
matching procedures and other methods to mitigate GvHD have not yet reached
a stage at which the transplantation of allogeneic marrow is a therapeutic
approach with an acceptably low risk.

Thus, it would seem that the creation of marrow banks is certainly not
imminent! However, since the immunological stumbling blocks may be overcome
in the near future and, since the occurrence of major calamities with
hundreds of radiation casualties can not be ruled out, it may be worthwhile
to speculate briefly on the organisation of future marrow banks. In principle, one could envisage two types of marrow banks which might be defined
as "individual" and "public" and which would supplement each other.

a) individual banks for the storage of autologous bone marrow would be
    created primarily as a precautionary measure for workers "at risk" in
    nuclear and space research and in nuclear industry (including repair
    crews, who are also at risk, albeit only during limited periods). For
    such individuals, the risk of fatal radiation exposure, although very
    low indeed, is considerably higher than that for the general popula-
    tion.

b) public banks for the storage of bone marrow from large numbers of
    selected volunteers. For logistic and ethical reasons (briefly outlined
    above) the establishment of such banks can hardly be expected in the
    very near future, unless the consequences of a major radiation accident
    lead to a drastic change of public opinion! The creation of public
    banks would also be facilitated if sufficient quantities of hemopoietic
    stem cells could be isolated from the peripheral blood, which would
    make the extraction of marrow under anesthesia unnecessary[a]. An alter-
    native approach would be using the autologous marrow samples already
    stored at the proposed individual banks. Such dual-purpose banks could
    of course provide preserved autologous marrow for those who donated the

----

[a] Fliedner and several other Euratom contractees (222-76-1 BIOD) are in
    fact investigating the feasibility of experimental banks for hemopoietic
    stem cells extracted from peripheral blood in the dog model (148, 149).

samples (thus serving as regular individual banks). Alternatively, the
marrow samples could, with the donors' permission, be used as allogeneic material for victims of radiation accidents who did not store
autologous marrow but do require a life-saving marrow graft.

If, for a moment, we accept the concept of public banks, the organization of such institutions could take place at a regional, national
or international level. Technical details, such as the methods of controlled freezing, the preparation and preservation of stem cell concentrates, regular checks for viability of the material in stock, etc.,
would need to be standardized and supervised by international bodies.
The operation of public banks would be somewhat similar to that of the
computerized organ exchange organizations which already exist and
function throughout the world (Eurotransplant, Scandiatransplant,
France-Transplant, etc.).

c) Desirability_and_feasibility. As mentioned above, the number of cases
(diseases or accidents) which have required bone marrow transplantation
has been rather limited in the past. Nevertheless, it might be useful
to already establish a few small regional banks at this time, in order
to acquire some practical experience in the selection of donors, the
effective storage of cells, the distribution and application of the
cellular material, etc. In fact, a large number of clinicians who prac-
tise human marrow transplantation today have indicated that the establishment of such seemingly futuristic marrow banks would be desirable.

Finally, an alternative approach to the described method of
marrow-banking should be mentioned. Dausset proposed in 1973 (150) that
lymphocytes (not marrow samples) of numerous volunteer donors should be
collected and stored. Large quantities of gradient-separated lymphocytes from all common HLA phenotypes should be preserved and all phenotypic (immunogenetic) data regarding the donors should be stored in a
computer. If a patient needed a marrow graft, phenotypically identical
lymphocyte samples would be retrieved from the bank and used for in
vitro cross-matching with the patient's cells (although obtaining
enough lymphocytes from an aplastic patient could be a problem; in such
cases, cells might be obtained from a lymph node biopsy). If an optimally matched volunteer donor was found, he or she would be invited to
come to the patient's location to donate the marrow. While this type of
banking would be relatively simple (since only lymphocytes need to be

preserved), the marrow donor might not always be available at the right time and place. Besides, determining optimal compatibility for marrow grafting by the simple cellular and serological techniques practised today (which indeed only require donor and recipient lymphocytes for in vitro typing and matching procedures) may not be adequate in the future.

In summary, establishing and operating "individual" banks should not create too many logistic problems, since the selection of optimal donor/recipient pairs would not be an integral part of the operation. However, the approach to "public" banking is different and requires also the intricate and somewhat risky collection of material from volunteers as well as optimal host/donor matching. In spite of the described logistic and ethical problems inherent to the creation of public marrow banks, some investigators (including the author of this review) would be in favor of establishing modest-sized public banks in the foreseeable future, according to the principles outlined above.

d) A few suggestions for the operation of a public marrow bank (highly schematic)

–   Collection and storage of donor samples. An intensive public campaign would be required to find a large number of volunteer marrow donors. Health checks of volunteer donors would have to be even more rigid than those applied for donors of conventional blood banks. Most importantly, individuals belonging to the "increased radiation hazard" group should be strongly encouraged not only to donate marrow for their own safety (see "individual banks") but to also act as volunteer donors for a public bank.

The quantity of marrow or stem cell concentrates to be collected and stored should be sufficient for at least one allogeneic transplant, preferably for several. Aspiration, preservation and storage of the material should be performed according to standardized methods. From the same donors, gradient-separated blood lymphocytes should also be collected and preserved in small aliquots for periodic updating of phenotypes (page 27) and for in vitro cross-matching); serum samples from the donors should also be collected and stored in small aliquots for similar purposes.

- <u>Storage of donor data</u>. All information on histocompatibility
antigens and other immunogenetic markers of the donor material
should be registered and stored in a regional computer. Eventually, several regional marrow banks might pool their information
in a national or international computerized storage and retrieval
system. The larger the pool of samples, the better the chance of
finding optimally matched allogeneic donors. The original data
will clearly require regular updating with regard to the donors'
addresses, health status, etc., as well as concerning newly dis-
covered immunogenetic markers that may be relevant for optimal
matching. The viability of the stored marrow or stem cell samples
should obviously also be checked at regular intervals.

- <u>Distribution of the stored material</u>. All relevant immunogenetic
information on the victim(s) of serious radiation accidents (who
may require a marrow transplant) should be collected and sent to
the public bank(s) at the earliest possible stage. The regional
or central computer should instantly retrieve donors who are
optimally matched for those immunogenetic markers which are considered most relevant to histocompatibility at that particular
time. Samples of the victim's blood or lymphocytes should then be
sent to the bank(s) where the most compatible donor(s) have been
spotted, in order to permit the performing of cross-matching procedures which are deemed necessary. Obviously, the stem cell
activity of the stored donor material will have to be checked in
vitro before considering the material as functional. It should
always be kept in mind that even optimally matched marrow from a
public bank will be from an unrelated allogeneic donor! Thus, at
the time of writing, the administration of such material is likely
to cause severe Graft versus Host Disease. Guidelines for a
decision as to whether or not to perform such a transplant and the
currently available methods to mitigate the expected GvHD, have
been presented on pages 36 to 41 and pages 61 to 63.

Acknowledgements

The author would like to express his deep gratitude to Dr. B. van der Kogel for substantial contributions to sections 2 and 3 of the manuscript and Dr. A.A. van Es for invaluable assistance in collecting essential references, especially those dealing with the case histories of the major radiation accidents (table III). Prof. D.W. van Bekkum as well as Drs. van der Kogel and van Es are gratefully acknowledged for carefully reading the manuscript (at various stages) and providing useful comments and criticism.

Ms D. v.d. Velden and Ms G.A. Bauer, who patiently typed the numerous versions of the manuscript and tables are most gratefully acknowledged. Mr. H.J. van Westbroek and the other members of the REP-Institutes' art department provided invaluable assistance in getting the more intricate tables into proper shape.

Dr. Lushbaugh of ERDA, Washington, kindly provided an updated listing of radiation accidents and Dr. Beninson and Mr. Holzer of UNSCEAR, Vienna were most helpful in collecting and providing publications with essential information.

References

1. Saenger, E.L.

     Radiation Accidents. The American Journal of Roentgenology,
     Radium Therapy and Nuclear Medicine, 84, 4 (1960), 715 - 728.

2. United Nations Scientific Committee on the Effects of Atomic Radiation.

     Report of the United Nations Scientific Committee on the Effects
     of Atomic Radiation. General Assembly document, 17th session,
     Suppl. No. 16 (A/5216). United Nations, N.Y., (1962).

3. Ougtherson, A.W. and Warren, S.

     Medical Effect of the Atomic Bomb in Japan. p. 477, McGraw-Hill,
     New York, (1956).

4. Andrews, A.A.

     Criticality accidents in Vinča, Yugoslavia and Oak Ridge,
     Tenessee. Comparison of radiation injuries and results of therapy.
     J. Am. Med. Ass. 179, (1962), 191 - 197.

5. Hempelmann, L.H., Lisco, H. and Hoffman, J.G.

     The acute radiation syndrome: A study of nine cases and a review
     of the problem. Ann. Ind. Med. 36, part 1, (1952), 279 - 510.

6. Gerstner, H.B.

     Acute radiation syndrome in man. US Armed Forces Med. J. 9,
     (1958), 313 - 354.

7. Operational Accidents and Radiation Exposure Experience within the
     United States Atomic Energy Commission 1943 - 1970. Division of
     Operational Safety. Washington D.C., 20545, issued fall 1971.

8. "Radiobiological basis for medical care following nuclear accidents".
     US Naval Medical Center, Bethesda, May 1970.

9. Brucer, M.

     The acute radiation syndrome. A medical report on the Y-12 acci-
     dent, June 16, (1958). USAEC report ORINS-25 (1959): v.e. United
     Nations document A/AC.82/G/L.270.

10. Institute of Nuclear Sciences "Boris Kidrich". Yugoslavian criticality
     accident, October 15, 1958. Nucleonics 17 (4), (1961), 106 - 156.

11. Paxton, H.C., Baker, R.D., Maraman, W.J. et al.

     Nuclear critical accident at the Los Alamos Scientific Laboratory
     on December 30, 1958. USAEC report LAMS-2293 (1959).

12. Howland, J.W., Ingram, M., Mermagen, H. et al.

    The Lockport incident: Accidental partial body exposure of humans to large doses of X-irradiation. In: Diagnosis and Treatment of Acute Radiation Injury. WHO, Geneva, (1961), 11 - 26.

13. Hasterlik, R.J., and Marinelli, L.D.

    Physical dosimetry and clinical observations involved in an accidental critical assembly excursion; Proc. 1st Int. Conf. Peaceful Uses Atomic Energy, Geneva 11, (1956), 25 - 34.

14. Van Bekkum, D.W. and De Vries, M.J.

    Radiation Chimaeras. Logos Press Book/Academic Press, London/New York (1967).

15. Mathé, G. and Schwarzenberg, L.

    Bone marrow transplantation in France 1958 - 1973. Transplantation Proc. VI, no. 4, (1974), 335 - 343.

16. Graw, R.G. and Herzig, G.P.

    Treatment of leukemia and aplastic anemia with histocompatible allogeneic bone marrow transplantation. Schweiz. med. Wschr. 102 (1972), 1573 - 1581.

17. Park, B.H., Biggar, W.D. and Good, R.A.

    Minnesota experience in bone-marrow transplantation in man, 1968 to June 1973. Transplantation Proc. VI, no. 4, (1974), 379 - 383.

18. Thomas, E.D., Storb, R., Clift, R.A. et al.

    Bone-marrow transplantation. New England J. Med. 292, part 1 and 2, (1975), 832 and 895.

19. Miller, D.G. and Diamond, H.D.

    The biological basis and clinical application of bone marrow transplantation. Med. Clinics N. America 45, (1961), 711 - 731.

20. McGovern, J.J., Russell, P.S., Atkins, L. and Webster, E.W.

    Treatment of terminal leukemic relapse by total-body irradiation and intravenous infusion of stored autologous bone marrow obtained during remission. New England J. Med. 260, (1959), 675 - 683.

21. Report of the United Nations Scientific Committee on the Effects of Atomic Radiation. General Assembly document, 24th session, Suppl. No. 13 (A7613). United Nations, N.Y. (1969).

22. Ionizing Radiation: Levels and Effects.

    A report of the United Nations Scientific Committee on the Effects of Atomic Radiation to the General Assembly.

    Volume I : Levels/Volume II: Effects. United Nations, N.Y., (1972).

70

23. Radiation Effects in Man: Early effects.

   Excerpt from: "Radiobiological Factors in Manned Space Flight"
   (W.H. Langham, editor). Report of the Space Radiation Study Panel
   of the Life Sciences Committee, Space Science Board. National
   Academy of Sciences, National Research Council, Washington DC
   (1967), 59 - 157.

24. Basic Radiation Protection Criteria.

   NCRP Report No. 39. NCRP Publications, PO Box 4867, Washington DC
   20008.

25. Storer, J.B., Harris, P.S., Furchner, J.E. and Langham, W.H.

   The relative biological effectiveness of various ionizing radiations in mammalian systems. Radiat. Res. 6, (1957), 188 - 288.

26. Broerse, J.J. and Barendsen, G.W.

   Relative biological effectiveness of fast neutrons for effects on
   normal tissues. Current topics in radiation research Quarterly 8,
   (1973), 305 - 350.

27. Rossi, H.H.

   Specification of Radiation Quality. Radiat. Res. 10, (1959), 522.

28. Barendsen, G.W., Beusker, T.L.J., Vergroesen, A.J. and Budke, L.

   Effects of different ionizing radiations on human cells in tissue
   culture. 1. Radiation techniques and dosimetry. Radiat. Res. 13,
   (1960), 832.

29. Elkind, M.M. and Sinclair, W.K.

   Recovery in X-irradiated mammalian cells.
   In: Current Topics in Radiation Research 1, (1965), 165 - 220.

30. Bergonié, J. and Tribondeau, L.

   Interprétation de quelques résultats de la radiothérapie et assai
   de fixation d'une technique rationelle. Comptes rendus Acad. Sci.,
   Paris, 143, (1906), 983 - 985.

31. Fabrikant, J.I.

   In: Radiobiology. Medical Publishers, Inc., Chicago (1972).

32. Elkind, M.M. and Whitmore, G.F.

   Radiobiology of cultured mammalian cells. N.Y. (1967). Gordon and
   Breach.

33. Wilson, B.R.

   Survival Studies of Whole-Body X-irradiated Germfree (Axenic) Mice.
   Radiat. Res. 20, (1963), 477 - 483.

34. Beninson, D., Placer, A. and Van der Elst, E.

   Estudio de un caso de irradiacion humane accidental. In: Handling
   of radiation accidents. May 1969, 415 - 429, WHO, Geneva (1969).

35. Hempelmann, L.A.

   The assessment of acute radiation injury. In: Diagnosis and treatment of acute radiation injury. p. 54, WHO, Geneva (1961).

36. Shipman, T.L.

   A radiation fatality resulting from massive overexposure to
   neutrons and gamma rays. In: Diagnosis and treatment of acute
   radiation injury. p. 113, WHO, Geneva (1961).

37. Brace, K.C. and Andrews, H.L.

   Early radiation death. Proc. 1st Int. Conf. Peaceful Uses Atomic
   Energy, Geneva 11, (1956), 115 - 117.

38. Mason, H.C., Mason, B.T. and Moss, W.S.

   Total-head (brain) X-irradiation of mice and primary factors
   involved. Brit. J. Radiol. 28, (1955), 495 - 507.

39. Hicks, S.P., Wright, K.A. and D'Amato, C.J.

   Time-intensity factors in radiation response. II. Some genetic
   factors in brain damage. Arch. Pathol. 66, (1958), 394 - 402.

40. Eldred, E. and Trowbridge, W.V.

   Neurological and EEG findings in the monkey after total body X-
   irradiation. Electroencephal. and Clin. Neurophysiol. 5, (1953),
   259 - 270.

41. Quastler, H.M.K. and Miller, A.M.

   Oral radiation death. Radiat. Res. 5, (1956), 338 - 353.

42. English, J.A.

   Localisation of radiation effects in rats' teeth. Oral Surg. Oral
   Med. Oral Pathol. 9, (1956), 1132 - 1138.

43. English, J.A., Wheatcroft, M.G. and Lyon, H.W.

   Longterm observations of radiation changes in salivary glands and
   the general effects of 1,000 r to 1,750 r of X-ray radiation
   locally administered to the heads of dogs. Oral Surg. Oral Med.
   Oral Pathol. 8, (1955), 87 - 99.

44. Cronkite, E.P. and Bond, V.P.

   Effects of radiation on mammals. Ann. Rev. Physiol. 18, (1956),
   483 - 526.

45. Bond, V.P., Silverman, M.S. and Cronkite, P.E.

    Pathogenesis and pathology of post-irradiation infection. Radiat. Res. 1, (1954), 389 - 400.

46. Quastler, H.

    The nature of intestinal radiation death. Radiat. Res. 4, (1956), 303 - 320.

47. Conard, R.A.

    Some effects of ionizing radiation on the physiology of the gas-tro-intestinal tract: A review. Radiat. Res. 5, (1956), 167 - 188.

48. Cairnie, A.B. and Millen, B.H.

    Fission of crypts in the small intestine of the irradiated mouse. Cell Tissue Kinet. 8, (1975), 189 - 196.

49. Conard, R.A., Cronkite, E.P., Brecher, G. and Strome, C.P.A.

    Experimental therapy of the gastro-intestinal syndrome produced by lethal doses of ionizing radiation. J. Appl. Physiol. 9, (1956), 227 - 233.

50. Delario, A.J.

    Roentgen Radium and Radioisotope Therapy. Lea and Febiger, Philadelphia, Pa., p. 112 (1953).

51. Sweet, R.D.

    Treatment of acute local radiation. Clinical Radiology 15, (1964), 55.

52. Schulz, E.H.

    Vorkommnisse und Strahlenunfälle in kerntechnischen Anlagen. Aus 20 Jahren internationaler Erfahrung. Verlag Karl Thiemig KG, München (1966).

53. TID-5360 (Suppl. 5)

    A summary of Industrial Accidents in USAEC facilities. United States Atomic Energy Commission. Technical Information Service, September (1959).

54. TID-5360 (Suppl. 2).

    A summary of Industrial Accidents in USAEC facilities 1963 - 1964. United States Atomic Energy Commission. Division of Technical Information, December 1965.

55. Handling of Radiation Accidents.

    Proceedings of a Symposium, Vienna, 19 - 23 May, 1969. IAEA, Vienna (1969).

56. Diagnosis and Treatment of Acute Radiation Injury.

Proc. of a Scientific Meeting jointly sponsored by the IAEA and
the WHO. Geneva, October 17 - 21, 1960.

57. Peaceful Uses of Atomic Energy

Proc. of the Intern. Conf. on the Peaceful Uses of Atomic Energy
Volume 11, Biological Effects of Radiation. Geneva, August 8 - 20,
1955. United Nations, New York (1956).

58. Bond, V.P., Fliedner, T.M. and Archambeau, J.O.

In: Mammalian Radiation Lethality. A disturbance in Cellular
Kinetics. Academic Press, New York, (1965).

59. Jammet, H., Mathé, G., Pendic, B., Duplan, J.F. et al.

Etude de six cas d'irradiation totale aigue accidentelle. Rev.
Franc. Etudes Clin. Biol. 4, (1959), 210 - 225.

60. Van der Waaij, D., De Vries, J.M. and Lekkerkerk, J.E.C.

Eliminating bacteria from monkeys with antibodies. In: Infections
and immunosuppression in subhuman primates. (ed. H. Balner and
W.I.B. Beveridge). Copenhagen, Munksgaard, (1970), 21 - 23.

61. United Nations Scientific Committee on the Effects of Atomic Radiation.
Report on the United Nations Scientific Committee on the Effects
of Atomic Radiation. General Assembly document, 17th session,
Suppl. no. 16 (A/5216). United Nations, N.Y., (1962), p. 174 and
175.

62. Jacobson, L.O., Simmons, E.L., Marks, E.K. et al.

The role of the spleen in radiation injury and recovery. J. Lab.
Clin. Med. 35, (1950), 746 - 770.

63. Lorenz, E., Uphoff, D., Reid, T.R. et al.

Modification of irradiation injury in mice and guinea pigs by
bone marrow injections. J. Natl. Cancer Inst. 12, (1951), 197 -
201.

64. Lindsley, D.L., Odell, T.T. and Tausche, F.G.

Implantation of functional erythropoietic elements following total-
body irradiation. Proc. Soc. Exp. Biol. Med. 90, (1955), 512 - 515.

65. Nowell, P.C., Cole, L.J., Habermeyer, J.G. et al.

Growth and continued function of rat marrow cells in X-radiated
mice. Cancer Res. 16, (1956), 258 - 261.

66. Mitchison, N.A.

The colonization of irradiated tissue by transplanted spleen cells.
Brit. J. Exp. Pathol. 37, (1956), 239 - 247.

74

67. Medawar, P.B.

Immunity to homologous grafted skin. II. The relationship between
the antigens of blood and skin. Brit. J. Exp. Pathol. 27, (1946),
15 - 24.

68. Hildeman, W.H.

Immunogenetics. Holden-Day, San Francisco, (1970).

69. Russell, P.S. and Monaco, A.P.

"The biology of tissue transplantation". Boston, (1965). Little,
Brown and Company.

70. Snell, G.D.

The H-2 locus of the mouse: observations and speculations concerning its comparative genetics and its polymorphism. Folia Biol.
14, (1968), 335 - 358.

71. Ivanyi, P.

The major histocompatibility antigens in various species. In:
Current topics in microbiology and immunology. 53, (1970),
14 - 24, Springer-Verlag, Berlin.

72. Klein, J., Bach, F.H., Festenstein, F., McDevitt, H.O., Schreffler,
D.C., Snell, G.D. and Stimpfling, J.H.

Genetic nomenclature for the H-2 complex of the mouse. Immunogenetics 1, (1974), 84.

73. Histocompatibility testing 1967.

(Report of a Conference and Workshop, Torino and Saint-Vincent,
Italy, June 1967) (eds. Curtoni, E.S., Mattiuz, P.L. and
Tosi, R.M.). Munksgaard, Copenhagen, Denmark.

74. Bach, F.H. and van Rood, J.J.

The major histocompatibility complex. Genetics and Biology. New
England J. Med. 295, (1976), 806-813, 872-878, 927-936.

75. Balner, H.

Current knowledge of the histocompatibility complex of rhesus
monkeys (A brief review). Transplantation Reviews 15, (1973),
50 - 61.

76. Vriesendorp, H.M.

Major histocompatibility complex of the dog. Thesis, Erasmus
University Rotterdam, December 1973. Bronder Offset B.V.,
Rotterdam (1973).

77. Balner, H.

Choice of animal species for modern transplantation research.
Transplantation Proc. VI, no. 4, (1974), 19 - 25.

78. Balner, H.

Genetic regions controlling immune responsiveness in primates.
Transplantation Proc. IX, no. 1, (1977), 837 - 845.

79. van Rood, J.J., van Leeuwen, A., Parlevliet, J., Termijtelen, A. and
Keuning, J.J.

LD typing by serology. IV. Description of the major locus with
three alleles. In: Histocompatibility testing. (Eds. Kissmeyer-
Nielsen, F., Svejgaard, A. and Thorsby, E.). Munksgaard,
Copenhagen, (1975), p. 629 - 636.

80. David, C.S., Shreffler, D.C. and Frelinger, J.A.

New lymphocyte antigen system (LNA) controlled by the Ir region
of the mouse H-2 complex. Proc. Nat. Acad. Sci. (Wash.) 70,
(1973), 2509 - 2514.

81. Transplantation Proceedings 1977.

Proceedings of the Sixth International Congress of the Transplantation Society, New York, 1976. Grune and Stratton, U.S.A.

82. Graw, R.G., Lohrman, H.P., Bull, M.I. et al.

Bone marrow transplantation following combination chemotherapy -
immunosuppression (BACT) in patients with acute leukemia. Transplantation Proc. VI, no. 4, (1974), 349 - 354.

83. Santos, G.W., Sensenbrenner, L.L., Burke, P.J., Mullins, G.M. et al.
Allogeneic marrow grafts in man using cyclophosphamide. Transplantation Proc. VI, no. 4, (1974), 345 - 348.

84. Ceppellini, R., Curtoni, E.S., Mattiuz, P.L., Miggiano, V.,
Scudeller, G. and Serra, A.

Genetics of leukocyte antigens: A family study of segregation and
linkage. Histocompatibility Testing 1967, (eds. Curtoni, E.S.,
Mattiuz, P.L. and Tosi, R.M.), Munksgaard, Copenhagen, Denmark.

85. Rood, J.J. van and Leeuwen, A. van.

Leukocyte grouping. A method and its application. J. Clin. Invest.
42, (1963), 1382 - 1390.

86. Bach, F.H. and Hirschhorn, K.

Lymphocyte interaction: A potential histocompatibility test in
vitro. Science 143, (1964), 813 - 814.

87. Rood, J.J. van, Leeuwen, A. van, Keunig, J.J. and van Oud Alblas, B.
    The serological recognition of the human MLC determinants using a
    modified cytotoxicity technique. Tissue Antigens 5, no. 2, (1975),
    73 - 79.

88. Balner, H. and Van Vreeswijk, W.
    The major histocompatibility complex of rhesus monkeys (RhL-A).
    V. Attempts at serological identification of MLR determinants
    and postulation of an I region in the RhL-A complex. Transplanta-
    tion Proc. VII, no. 1, (1975), p. 13 - 20.

89. Koch, C.T., Van Hooff, J.P., Van Leeuwen, A. et al.
    The relative importance of matching for the MLC versus the HL-A
    loci in organ transplantation. Histocompatibility Testing (1972),
    (eds. Dausset, J. and Colombani, J.), 521 - 524.

90. van Es, A.A., Marquet, R.L., van Vreeswijk, W., Tank, B. and Balner, H.
    Influence of matching for RhLA (SD) antigens and of mixed lympho-
    cyte reactivity on allograft survival in unrelated rhesus monkeys.
    Transplantation Proc. IX, no. 1, (1977), 257 - 260.

91. McDevitt, H.O. and Benacerraf, B.
    Genetic control of specific immune response. Advance in Immunology
    11, no. 31, (1969), 31 - 74.

92. Cudkowicz, G.
    Peculiar immunobiology of bone marrow allografts. I. Graft rejec-
    tion by irradiated responder mice. J. Exp. Med. 134, (1971), 83.

93. Uphoff, D.E.
    Genetic factors influencing irradiation protection by bone marrow.
    III. Midlethal irradiation of inbred mice. J. Nat. Cancer Inst.
    30, (1963), 1115 - 1151.

94. Balner, H., de Vries, M.J. and van Bekkum, D.W.
    Secondary disease in rat radiation chimeras. J. Nat. Cancer Inst.
    32, no. 2, (1964), 419 - 459.

95. Van Bekkum D.W.
    Chapter 29: Experimental basis for the therapy of radiation injury
    to the haemopoietic system. In: Technical reports series no. 123
    "Manual on Radiation Haematology". International Atomic Energy
    Agency, Vienna, (1971).

96. Van Bekkum, D.W., Vos, O. and Weyzen, W.W.H.
    Homo- et hétérogreffe tissus hematopoiétiques chez la souris.
    Rve. d'Hémat. II, (1956), 477 - 485.

77

97. Van Putten, L.M., Van Bekkum, D.W., De Vries, M.J. and Balner, H.
    The effect of preceding blood transfusions on the fate of homo-
    logous bone marrow grafts in lethally irradiated monkeys. Blood
    30, no. 6, (1967), 749 - 757.

98. De Vries, M.J., Crouch, B.G., Van Putten, L.M. and Van Bekkum, D.W.
    Pathologic changes in irradiated monkeys treated with bone marrow.
    J. Nat. Cancer Inst. 27, (1961), 67 - 97.

99. Dicke, K.A. and Van Bekkum, D.W.
    Avoidance of acute secondary disease by purification of hemo-
    poietic stem cells with density gradient centrifugation. Exp.
    hematol. 20, (1970), 126.

100. Epstein. R.B., Bryant, J. and Thomas, E.D.
    Cytogenetic demonstration of permanent tolerance in adult outbred
    dogs. Transplantation 5, no. 2, (1967), 267 - 272.

101. Storb, R., Kolb, H.J., Graham, T.C. et al.
    Treatment of established graft-versus-host disease in dogs by
    anti-thymocyte serum or prednisone. Blood 42, (1973), 601 - 609.

102. Vriesendorp, H.M., Zurcher, C., Bull, R.W., Los, W.R.T.,
    Meera Khan, P., Van de Tweel, J.G., Zweibaum, A. and Van Bekkum, D.W.
    Take and Graft versus Host reactions of allogeneic bone marrow in
    tissue-typed dogs. Transplantation Proc. VII, no. 1, (1975),
    849 - 853.

103. Mathé, G., Bernard, J., De Vries, M.J., Schwarzenberg, L.,
    Larrieu, M.J., Lalanne, C.M., Dutreix, A., Amiel, J.L. and Surmont, J.
    Nouveaux essais de greffe de moelle osseuse homologue après
    irradiation totale chez des enfants atteints de leucémie aiguë en
    rémission. Le problème du syndrome secondaire chez l'homme. Rev.
    Hématol. 15, (1960), 115 - 161.

104. Schwartz, R.S. and Beldotti, L.
    Malignant lymphomas following allogeneic disease: Transition from
    an immunological to a neoplastic disorder. Science 149, (1965),
    1511.

105. Mathé, G., Amiel, J.L., Schwarzenberg, L., Cattan, A., et al.
    Successful allogeneic bone marrow transplantation in man:
    chimerism, induced specific tolerance and possible antileukemic
    effects. Blood 25, (1965), 179 - 196.

106. Storb, R., Rudolph, R.H., Kolb, H.J. et al.

   Marrow grafts between DL-A matched caninen littermates. Transplantation 15, (1973), 92 - 100.

107. Vriesendorp, H.M., Bijnen, A.B., Zürcher, C. and van Bekkum, D.W.

   Donor selection and bone marrow transplantation in dogs. Histocompatibility Testing 1975, (ed. Kissmeyer-Nielsen, F.),
   Munksgaard, Copenhagen, Denmark, p. 963 - 91.

108. Schaefer, U.W.

   Personal communication.

109. Neefe, J.R., Merritt, C.B., Darrow, C.C., and Rogentine, G.N.

   Beneficial influence of limited histocompatibility of bone marrow
   grafted to unrelated rhesus monkeys preconditioned with X-ray and
   ALS. Transplantation Proc. VI, no. 2, (1974), 125 - 128.

110. Annual Report 1976.

   REP Institutes of the Organization for Health Research TNO,
   Rijswijk (ZH), The Netherlands.

111. Livnat, S., Klein, J., Bach, F.H.

   Graft versus host reaction in strains of mice identical for H-2K
   and H-2D antigens. Nature New Biol. 243, (1973), 42.

112. Klein, J. and Park, J.M.

   Graft versus host reaction across different regions of the H-2
   complex of the mouse. J. Exp. Med. 137, (1973), 1213.

113. Dausset, J.

   Proposal for a World Bank of Reactive Cells from Bone Marrow.
   Transplantation Proc. VI, no. 4, (1974), 429 - 430.

114. Van Bekkum, D.W.

   The double barrier in bone marrow transplantation. Seminars in
   Hematology 11, no. 3, (1974), 325 - 340.

115. Uphoff, D.E.

   Preclusion of secondary phase of irradiation syndrome by inocula-
   tion of fetal hematopoietic tissue following lethal total body X-
   irradiation. J. Nat. Cancer Inst. 20, (1958), 625 - 632.

116. Crouch, B.G.

   Transplantation of fetal hemopoietic tissues into irradiated mice
   and rats. Proc. 7th Congr. Europ. Soc. Haemat., London, 1959,
   973 - 978, (1960).

117. Van Bekkum, D.W.

   Prevention and control of secondary disease following allogeneic
   bone marrow transplantation. From: "Bone marrow conservation,
   culture and transplantation", IAEA, Vienna, Austria (1969).

118. Amiel, J.G. and Mathé, G.

   A comparison of the sensitivity to storage at 37° C in Tyrode
   solution of immunologically competent cells and of myeloid cells.
   Nature 200, (1963), 1224 - 1225.

119. Van Bekkum, D.W., Ledney, G.D., Balner, H., Van Putten, L.M. and
   De Vries, M.J.

   Suppression of secondary disease following foreign bone marrow
   grafting with antilymphocyte serum. Antilymphocytic Serum. Ciba
   Foundation Study Group no. 29, (1967), p. 97, Churchill, London.

120. Cosgrove, G.E., Upton, A.C., Popp, R.A. and Congdon, C.C.

   Inhibition of foreign spleen reaction by inactivation of donor
   cells with recipient antigen. Proc. Soc. Exp. Biol. Med. 102,
   (1959), 525 - 527.

121. In vitro Culture of Hemopoietic Cells.

   Proc. Worksh./Symp. on: In vitro culture of hemopoietic cells.
   Radiobiological Institute TNO, Rijswijk, Sept.-Oct. 1971. (eds.
   D.W. van Bekkum and K.A. Dicke). Publ. Radiobiological Institute
   TNO, Rijswijk (ZH), (1972).

122. Dicke, K.A., Van Hooft, J.I.M. and Van Bekkum, D.W.

   The selective elimination of immunologically competent cells from
   bone marrow and lymphatic cell mixtures. II. Mouse spleen cell
   fractionation on a discontinuous albumin gradient. Transplantation
   6, (1968), 562.

123. Dicke, K.A., Platenburg, M.G.C. and Van Bekkum, D.W.

   Colony formation in agar: in vitro assay for haemopoietic stem
   cells. Cell Tiss. Kinet. 4, (1971), 463.

124. Schaefer, U.W., Dicke, K.A. and Van Bekkum, D.W.

   Recovery of haemopoiesis in lethally irradiated monkeys by frozen
   allogeneic bone marrow grafts. Rev. Europ. Etudes Clin. et Biol.
   XVII, (1972), 483 -488,

125. Dicke, K.A., Schaefer, U.W. and Van Bekkum, D.W.

   Allogeneic bone marrow transplantation in man. Strahlen, Blutge-
   rinnen und Hämostase. XVI. Hamburger Symp. über Blutgerinnung, 1
   und 2 Juni 1973. F.K. Schattauer Verlag, Stuttgart, (1974).

126. Löwenberg, B., de Zeeuw, H.M.C., Dicke, K.A. and van Bekkum, D.W.
    Nature of the graft versus host reactivity of fetal liver cell
    transplants in mice. J. Nat. Cancer Inst. 58, (1977), 959.

127. Van Bekkum, D.W. and Streilen, W.
    Workshop on Bone Marrow Transplantation. Transplantation Proc. IV,
    no. 1, (1973), 997 - 999.

128. Thierfelder, S. and Rodt, H.
    Host versus theta graft reactions. Exp. Hematol. suppl. 4, (1976),
    165.

129. Batchelor, J.R. and Howard, J.G.
    Synergic and antagonistic effects of isoantibody upon graft-versus
    host disease. Transplantation 3, (1965), 161.

130. van Bekkum, D.W.
    Bone marrow transplantation. Transplantation Proc. IX, no. 1,
    (1977), 147 - 154.

131. van Bekkum, D.W., Roodenburg, J, Heidt, P.J. and Van der Waaij, D.
    Mitigation of secondary disease of allogeneic mouse radiation
    chimeras by modification of the intestinal microflora. J. Natl.
    Cancer Inst. 52, (1974), 401 - 404.

132. Pillow, R.P., Epstein, R.B., Buckner, C.D. et al.
    Treatment of marrow failure by isogeneic marrow infusion. New
    England J. Med. 275, (1966), 94 - 97.

133. Hurst, G.S., Ritchie, R.H.
    In: Radiation accidents: dosimetric aspects of neutron and gamma
    ray exposures. Oak Ridge, Oak Ridge National Laboratory (ORNL-
    2748 A), 12, (1959).

134. Auxier, J.A.
    Dosimetric considerations in critically exposures. In: Diagnosis
    and treatment of acute radiation injury. WHO, Geneva, (1961),
    141 - 150.

135. Bone marrow transplantation from histocompatible, allogeneic donors
    for aplastic anemia. Prepared by the Advisory Committee of the
    Bone Marrow Transplant Registry. JAMA vol. 236, 10 (1976), 1131 -
    1135.

136. Storb, R., Thomas, E.D., Weiden, P.L. et al.
    Aplastic anemia treated by allogeneic bone marrow transplantation:
    a report on 49 new cases from Seattle. Blood, vol. 48, 6, (1976),
    817 - 841.

137. Camitta, B.M., Thomas, E.D., Nathan, D.G., Santos, G., Gordon-Smith, E.C., and Gale, R.P.

   Severe aplastic anemia: a prospective study of the effect of early marrow transplantation on acute mortality. Blood 48, (1976), 48 - 63.

138. Storb, R., Gluckman, E., Thomas, E.D. et al.

   Treatment of established human graft versus host disease by anti-thymocyte globulin. Blood 44, (1974), 57 - 75.

139. Van Bekkum, D.W.

   Strategy of clinical bone marrow transplantation with emphasis on treatment of combined immune deficiency. Transplantation Proc. VI, no. 4, (1974), 373 - 377.

140. Doorn, L.J.

   Behandlung Immunologischer Defektzustände. Helv. Ped. Acta suppl. 3 (1975).

141. Bortin, M.M. and Rimm, A.A.

   Severe combined immunodeficiency disease: characterization of the disease and results of transplantation. Transplantation Proc. IX, no. 1, (1977), 169 - 170.

142. Diagnosis and Treatment of Incorporated Radionuclides.

   Proceedings of a seminar, Vienna 8-12 December, 1975 organized by the IAEA (International Atomic Energy Agency) and WHO (World Health Organization). IAEA (1976).

143. Faires, R.A. and B.H. Parks

   Radioisotope laboratory techniques. Newness, London (1960).

144. Nack, P., Arndt, D., Schüttmann.

   Organizational forms of medical care in case of radiation accidents in the GDR. From: Proceedings International Symposium on the handling of radiation accidents, IAEA, Vienna, Austria (1977).

145. Bresson, G. and Nénot, J.C.

   Moyens mis en oeuvre en cas d'accident radiologique. From: Proceedings International Symposium on the handling of radiation accidents, IAEA, Vienna, Austria (1977).

146. Fliedner, T.M.

   Organizational aspects of the handling of radiation accidents in the federal republic of Germany. From: Proceedings International Symposium on the handling of radiation accidents, IAEA, Vienna, Austria (1977).

82

147. Linnemann, R.E. and Mettler, F.A.

Emergency medical assistance programs for nuclear power reactors.
From: Proceedings International Symposium on the handling of
radiation accidents, IAEA, Vienna, Austria (1977).

148. Fliedner, T.M., Flad, H.D., Bruch, Ch. et al.

Treatment of aplastic anemia by blood stem cell transfusion: a
canine model. Haematologica, vol. 61, 141, (1976), 141 - 156.

149. Flad, H.D., Krumbacher, K., Schnappauf, W. et al.

Transplantation of allogeneic dog leukocytes into lethally irradiated matched or mismatched recipients. Zeitschr. für Immuni-
tätsforschung - Immunbiology, Bd. 152, (1976), 326 - 330.

150. Dausset, J.

Proposal for a world bank of reactive cells from bone marrow.
Transplantation Proc. VI, no. 4, (1974), 429 - 430.

131. Quastler, H., Lanzl, E.F., Keller, M.E. and Osborne, J.W.

Acute intestinal radiation death. III. Studies in röntgen death
in mice. Am. J. Physiol. 164, (1951), 546.

152. Cronkite, E.P.

The diagnosis, prognosis and treatment of radiation injuries produced by atomic bombs. Radiology 56, (1951), 661 - 669.

153. Rajewski, B., Heuse, O. and Aurand, K.

Weitere untersuchungen zum Problem der Ganzkorper-Bestrahlung der
weissen Maus. Sofortiger Tod durch Strahlung. Zeitschrift Naturf.
86, (1953), 157 - 159.

154. Pickering, J.E., Langham, W.H. and Rambach, W.A.

The effects from massive doses of high dose rate gamma radiation
on monkeys. USAF School of Aviation Medicine, Report no. 55 - 77,
(1955).